Strawberry benefits: know them

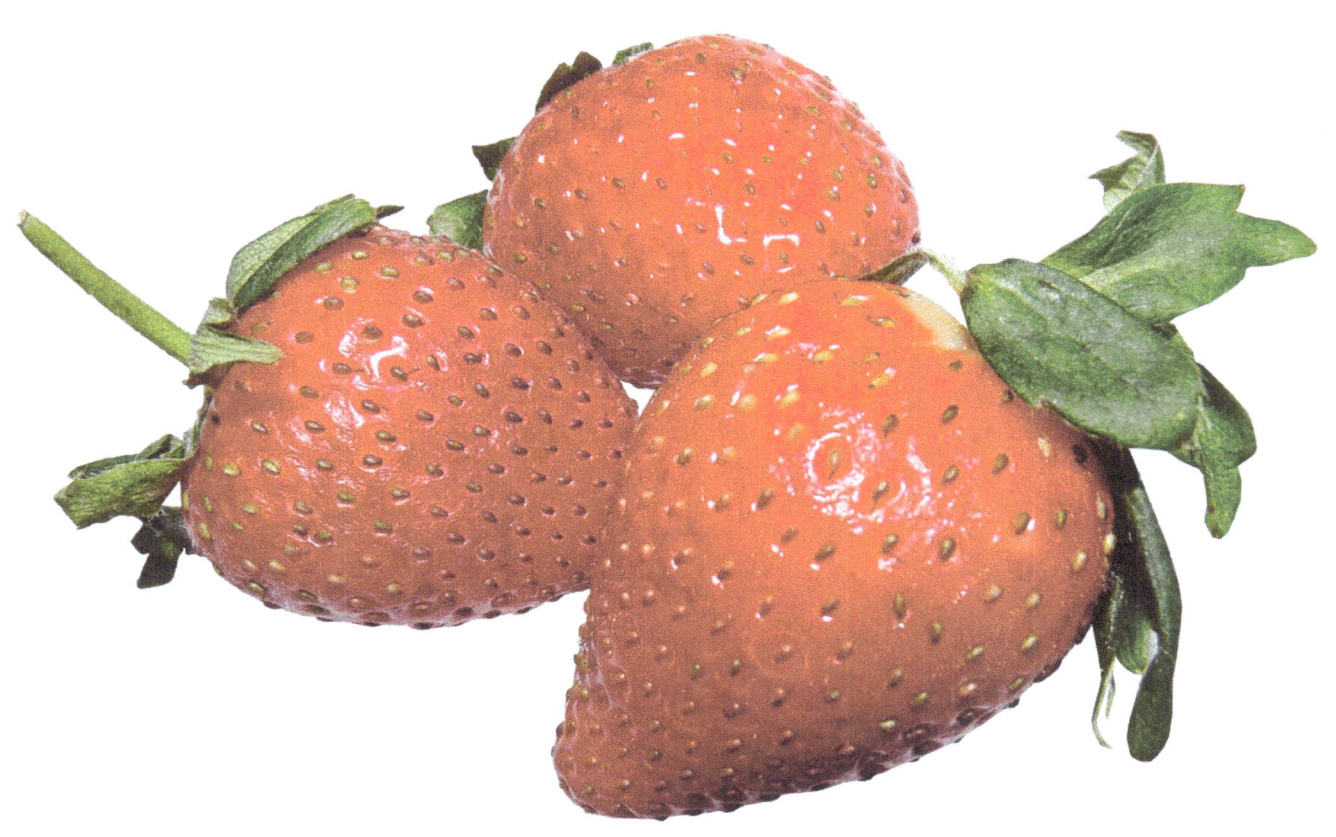

Strawberry benefits: know them

Are you a fan of strawberry fruits? If you give your body many benefits, as the benefits of strawberries are very numerous and amazing, follow the article to learn about these benefits.

Strawberry benefits: know them

In the following, let us learn about the benefits of strawberries and how to eat them, in addition to knowing their potential harms:

The benefits of strawberries

The potential benefits of strawberries are as follows:

1. Increase the strength of the immune system

Strawberries contain a good percentage of vitamin C, and this vitamin is able to enhance and strengthen the health of the immune system, and it works to make the digestive system absorb iron better, and this reduces the incidence of iron deficiency anemia.

2. Support the work of the digestive system

The phosphorous present in strawberries contributes to improving the digestive process, as it provides the body with energy.

3. Contribute to reducing the incidence of cancer

Strawberries are rich in antioxidants that fight free radicals, and in this sense, strawberries may have a role in reducing the incidence of cancer.

4. Regulating blood sugar levels

One of the most prominent benefits of strawberries is that they may contribute to regulating sugar levels in the body, due to the fact that they contain dietary fibers that contribute to reducing the feeling of hunger, and therefore eating less food, and this contributes to regulating blood sugar.

5. Promote cardiovascular health

One of the benefits of strawberries is to enhance and improve the health of the heart and arteries in general, and this potential benefit is attributed to the fact that strawberries contain all of the following:

Fiber that may help lower levels of bad cholesterol in the body.
Potassium: Potassium promotes the health of blood vessels, and prevents high blood pressure, and this leads to the promotion of heart health
Moderate levels of folic acid, which helps improve heart health.
Antioxidants, such as: anthocyanin, and anti-inflammatory, such as: flavonoids, which all help reduce the chances of heart disease.

6. Contribute to weight reduction

Strawberries are good for weight loss diets, for the following two reasons:

Strawberries contain dietary fibers that reduce the feeling of hunger and this was mentioned earlier.
Strawberries have few calories, as every 100 grams of fresh strawberries contains only 32 calories.

7. Extension of the body with many nutrients

Strawberries are a good source of vitamin K, manganese, folic acid, potassium, B vitamins, copper, magnesium, and omega-3, all of which are important for a healthy body.

How to eat strawberries

To obtain the benefits of strawberries, it is necessary to know the ways to eat them, and the following are the most prominent of these methods:

Eat fresh strawberries directly.

Prepare strawberry juice, which can be combined with many fruits, such as: bananas, and in this way can ensure more health benefits for the body.

Put strawberry slices with salads, especially strawberries, which have a sour taste.

Making strawberry jam, but it should be noted that this method will make the body get huge amounts of sugar, which it is indispensable.

Strawberry side effects

Despite the benefits of strawberries, they may cause some potential harm to some, the most prominent of which are the following:

1. Allergy

For sensitive people, strawberries can cause severe allergic reactions.

Symptoms of an allergic attack include: swelling, redness of the mouth, lips and tongue, eczema, rash, headache, runny nose and itchy eyes.

If an allergy is suspected, it is recommended to avoid eating this fruit.

2. Slow blood clotting

Eating large quantities of strawberries may slow blood clotting when injured, and this is due to the ability of strawberries to increase blood fluidity.

3. Gastrointestinal disorders

Strawberries can cause stomach cramps for some, and they may also be the main cause of diarrhea, and this happens if you eat very large amounts of them.

Learn about the benefits of strawberries for the blood

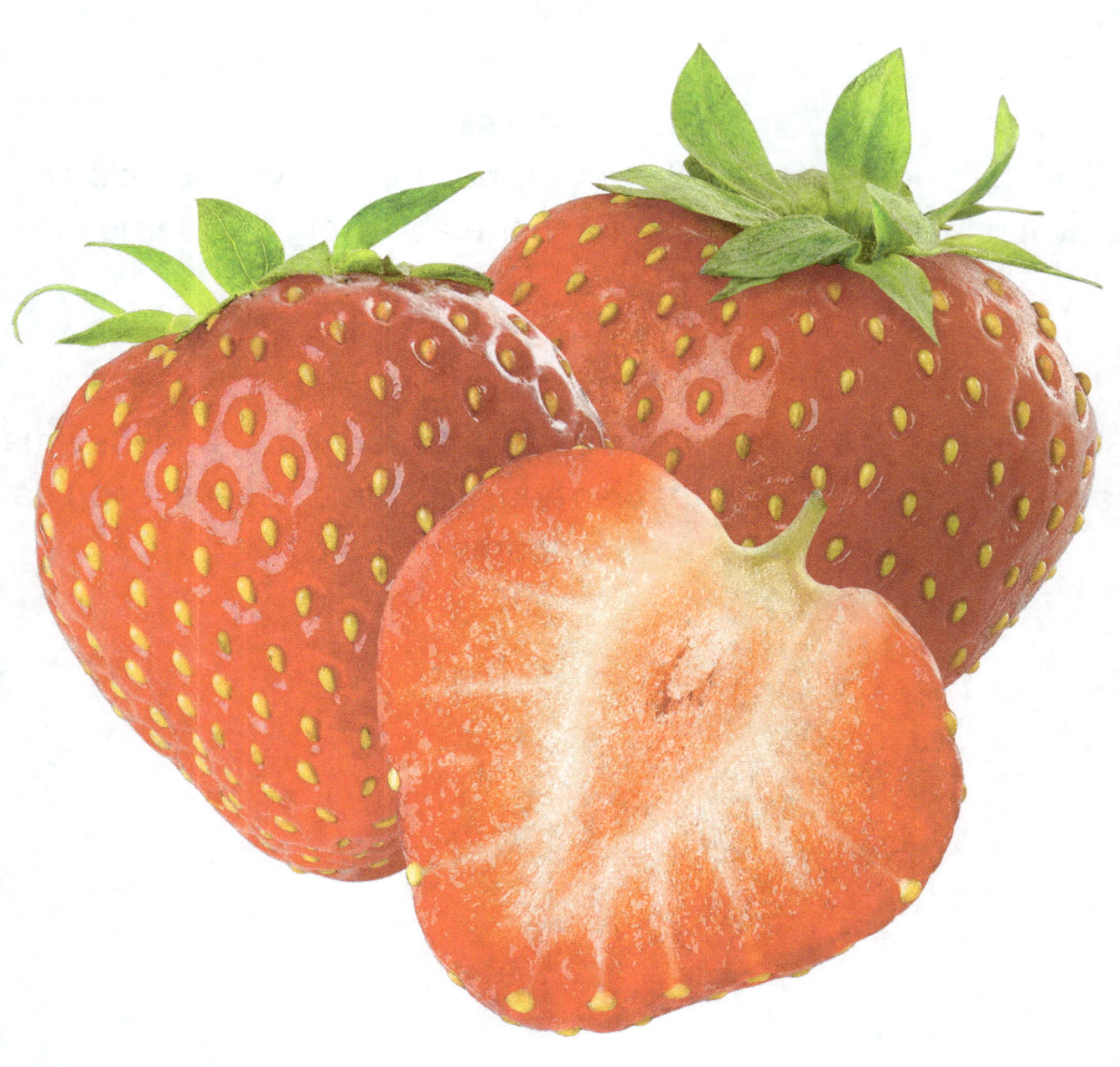

Learn about the benefits of strawberries for the blood

The benefits of strawberries for the blood and the body are many and varied, so what are the most important of these benefits of strawberries for the blood in particular, and what are its other benefits? The answers and more can be found in the article.

Learn about the benefits of strawberries for the blood

Let's get acquainted with the following about the benefits of strawberries for the blood and the body, and the most important information related to this delicious fruit:

Benefits of strawberries for the blood and circulatory system

Here is a list of the most important potential benefits of strawberries for the blood and circulatory system:

1. Improve the absorption of iron from food

Eating fresh strawberries regularly may improve the digestive system's ability to absorb and benefit from iron from food and supplements.

The potential benefits of strawberries in this regard are due to the richness of this delicious fruit in vitamin C, as vitamin C is one of the nutrients that helps to enhance the absorption of iron in the body.

2. Regulating blood pressure levels

Eating strawberries may help regulate blood pressure and keep it under control as much as possible, often for the following reasons:

Strawberries contain a relatively high amount of potassium, as potassium deficiency increases the chances of developing high blood pressure.

Strawberries are rich in anthocyanin, a type of powerful antioxidant that may help dilate blood vessels and reduce the chances of high blood pressure.

So, in the long run, eating strawberries may help protect against many cardiovascular diseases, especially diseases that may be caused by high blood pressure.

3. Promote heart health

One of the benefits of strawberries for the blood and the circulatory system is its potential ability to improve the health of the heart and arteries in general, and the potential benefits of strawberries in this regard are attributed to the following:

Strawberries contain fiber that may help reduce bad cholesterol levels in the body.

Strawberries contain moderate amounts of folic acid, which helps improve heart health.

Strawberries are rich in many important nutrients and substances that help reduce the chances of developing heart and circulatory diseases, especially the following: antioxidants and anti-inflammatory.

4. Other blood benefits of strawberries

The benefits of strawberries for the blood are not limited to what was mentioned above, but in the following are some of the other benefits of strawberries for the blood and the circulatory system:

Ensuring the proper and healthy occurrence of blood clotting processes in the body, and reducing the chances of developing blood clots.

Strengthen and improve blood circulation in the brain.

Improving the ability of blood cells to resist harmful oxidative processes.

Other benefits of strawberries for the body

In addition to the benefits of strawberries for the blood and circulatory system, strawberries may have many other health benefits, most notably:

Reducing the chances of developing cancer, especially the following types of cancer: colon cancer and esophageal cancer.
Strengthen the body's immunity, and improve its ability to resist various types of diseases and infections.
Losing excess weight and resisting obesity. And
Improving the health and appearance of the skin, and protecting against the signs of aging or delaying the appearance of the skin.
Improve brain health, and slow the rate of memory loss and deterioration that may arise with normal ageing. And
Regulating blood sugar levels, which may help keep diabetes under control.
Reducing pain that may accompany diseases, such as: arthritis, gout.
Improving the health of the pregnancy, and reducing the chances of fetal malformations and birth defects.
Regulating digestion and resisting constipation.
Stop hair loss.
Increased sperm count.
Teeth whitening.
-Maintain eye health

strawberry nutritional value

The benefits of strawberries for the blood, the circulatory system and the whole body result from its high nutritional value, as each 100 grams of fresh strawberries contains the following:

Nutrient value Nutritional value
Energy 32 calories
Water 90.95 g
Proteins 0.67 g
Dietary fiber 2 grams
Calcium 16 milligrams
Iron 0.41 milligrams
Magnesium 13 milligrams
Phosphorous 24 milligrams
Potassium 153 milligrams
Zinc 0.14 milligrams
Selenium 0.4 mcg
Vitamin C 58.8 milligrams
Vitamin B6 0.05 mg
Folate 24 mcg

Strawberry side effects

Despite the benefits of strawberries for the blood and various body systems, eating strawberries may cause many damage and health complications at times, such as:

1. Strawberry allergy

Symptoms of strawberry allergy may appear, and these symptoms often appear on the affected person within a period ranging from 5-15 minutes after eating strawberries, and these symptoms include:

rash.

Itchy skin.

Change in skin color.

Swallowing difficulties.

Swelling in the mouth or tongue.

2. Effect on sugar levels

Strawberries provide the body with a high dose of sugar, especially when eating large amounts of it, and this negatively affects especially diabetics.

3. Exposure to other health complications

You can experience more other complications despite the benefits of strawberries for the blood and the body as a whole, the most prominent of which are the following:

Possible health complications for people with health problems or kidney disease.

Increased blood fluidity, which may cause an increase in the chances of bleeding and bruising, so it is preferable to avoid eating strawberries by the following groups:

People with hemorrhagic diseases.

.Patients about to undergo surgery

What are the benefits of strawberry for teeth?

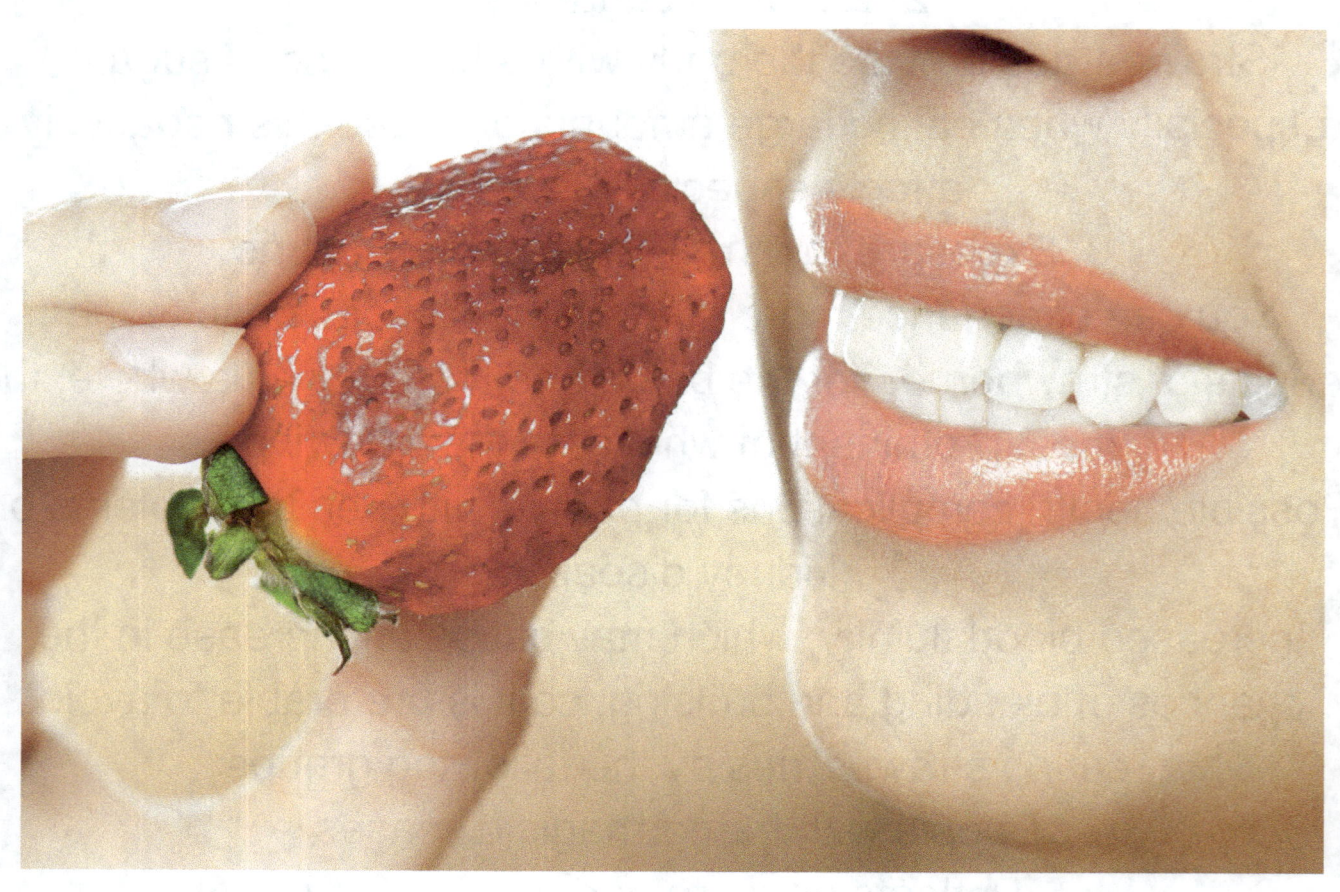

What are the benefits of strawberry for teeth?
Recently, many recipes aimed at whitening teeth have spread, most notably recipes containing strawberries, here are the most prominent benefits of strawberries for teeth.

What are the benefits of strawberry for teeth?
strawberry
Benefits of strawberry for teeth
Strawberries are good for your overall health and also for your teeth. Here are the most prominent dental benefits of strawberries:
Using strawberries and rubbing the teeth with them leads to teeth whitening, because they contain malic acid, which is a natural whitener for the enamel of the teeth and helps lighten the smile.
Strawberries are full of minerals, nutrients and vitamins, especially vitamin C, which is necessary to maintain healthy gums, as only one serving, about eight strawberries, provides vitamin C at a rate that exceeds the percentage of vitamin C in oranges.
How can you get the benefits of strawberry for the teeth?
To take advantage of all the benefits of strawberries for the teeth, we advise you to eat fresh strawberries and eat them directly, so that you will get all their benefits at the level of teeth and at the level of general health as well.
Also, rubbing your teeth with it can help you get the aforementioned benefits.

Benefits of strawberry for teeth

Although there are many benefits of strawberry for the teeth, there are a lot of harms that may happen to you when you overuse it, namely:

Strawberries are highly acidic, and using them frequently in dental recipes can damage your teeth. Because the severity of acidity may lead to the erosion of the tooth enamel, and the enamel of the teeth, once eaten, cannot be regenerated.

The bleaching resulting from the use of strawberries is not real bleaching, it is only superficial bleaching, as the malic acid helps to remove plaque and pigmentation from the teeth, which gives a whiter smile, but in fact it is not real bleaching of the tooth. About an hour, and after a short period of time, your teeth will return to the way they were, as the effect is considered superficial.

Strawberries are full of natural sugar. Placing strawberry or strawberry juice on the teeth may increase the chances of developing tooth decay.

Other benefits of strawberries

Here are the main benefits of strawberries for your overall health:

Strawberries maintain heart health and protect against the risk of heart attacks, because of their role in lowering blood pressure and increasing good cholesterol.

Strawberries protect against the risk of cancer, as they have many anti-cancer effects.

Strawberries help in reducing the disorders associated with obesity, diabetes and bacterial diseases.

Tips for maintaining healthy teeth and gums

Here are some tips you can do to keep your teeth healthy:

Maintaining tooth brushing: and sticking to it at least twice a day, as it contributes to maintaining the health of teeth and gums and reducing the risk of cavities.

Use dental products that contain fluoride: Fluoride helps protect teeth from decay and is a common ingredient in toothpastes and mouthwashes.

Flossing at least once a day: Flossing helps remove plaque and bacteria from between the teeth, especially those that the toothbrush cannot reach or remove.

Visit the dentist regularly: Regular visits to the dentist help diagnose and solve dental problems before they get worse.

Stay away from smoking: Smoking affects the teeth and gums, as it leads to yellowing of the teeth and the appearance of bad breath and is a risk factor for gum disease.

Use of mouthwash: Mouthwash helps treat dental problems, maintains oral hygiene, and contributes to solving the problem of bad breath, but it is not a substitute and cannot replace flossing and brushing.

Reduce sugary foods and starches: Consuming and eating large amounts of sugar increases the risk of tooth decay.

Stay away from soft drinks and sugar-sweetened drinks: You can replace them with drinking water and drinking unsweetened drinks, and if you drink sugar-sweetened drinks, eat them only in small quantities.

Maintaining teeth: healthy habits to stick to

Do you want to preserve teeth for a longer period? Here are some healthy habits in order to maintain the health and safety of teeth.

Maintaining teeth: healthy habits to stick to

Maintaining dental health usually requires following a set of healthy daily habits that have an important role in its safety. Here are the most prominent healthy habits that contribute to preserving teeth and protecting them from decay and various other diseases:

Teeth preservation methods

There are many healthy habits and ways to maintain teeth, and the most prominent of these healthy habits that help maintain teeth are the following:

1. Use flossing and mouthwash

In the event that you are not one of those who brush their teeth properly and only use the brush and paste, it certainly will not help you reduce your risk of tooth decay and gum disease. Using floss and mouthwash in addition to the appropriate brush and paste is the best way to ensure that the way you care for your teeth is correct.

Therefore, be sure to use mouthwash in particular along with the daily dental cleaning process, at least twice per day, to ensure that the cleaning process reaches 100% of the oral cavity.

This protects yourself from oral and dental problems, fights gum infections and bad breath, and it has been found that the use of lotion may help reduce the accumulation of plaque more than using a toothbrush and flossing only.

2. Use a soft toothbrush

It is usually recommended to use a small brush with soft bristles wet with water, and to stay away from hard, dry toothbrushes that may cause enamel erosion over time and injure the gums, which may make your teeth weak and yellow.

We also advise you to always rinse your toothbrush with lukewarm water to soften it before using it.

3. Eat healthy snacks

If you eat 3 meals a day, make sure that they are low in carbohydrates and simple sugars that may harm your teeth, and try to avoid as much as possible a large number of snacks and snacks during the day, especially those that contain high levels of sugar and unhealthy, such as: juices, drinks Invasive.

4. Avoid smoking

Smoking is a bad habit that harms all parts of your body, but it may be one of the most bad habits for the health of your teeth and gums. Smoking reduces blood flow to your mouth, which may increase the chances of gum disease and oral cancer.

It may also cause discoloration and yellowing of the teeth, and the occurrence of bad odor, not only that, but if you are receiving dental treatment or undergoing oral surgery, smoking may slow down the healing process.

5. Visit the dentist regularly

Many people may not want to visit the dentist, because they are afraid of the pain or injections that may accompany this visit, but if you want to prevent yourself from this suffering, you must get used to yourself and your children to repeat this visit on a regular basis.

6. Eating gum

We may encourage you to make the habit of chewing gum from time to time, at least once a day, and here we mean sugar-free gum, which may enhance the process of saliva secretion in the mouth, and reduce its dryness, which may increase the possibility of germs multiplying in the mouth.

7. Use a straw or straw

Of course, we do not advise you to drink any of the soft drinks or that contain soda that may harm your teeth, but here we will give you another important advice, which is to make sure to use the straw when consuming any of the sour drinks or the abundance of which may harm your teeth, such as: citrus drinks or sweetened juices.

This will reduce the chances of enamel erosion due to acid, or tooth decay due to sugars.

8. Change your toothbrush regularly

Changing the toothbrush periodically is important in order to maintain the teeth and the health of the gums in general, as the toothbrush must be changed every 3 months; This is because after this period it becomes ineffective and polluted.

Teeth whitening with strawberries: an effective recipe?

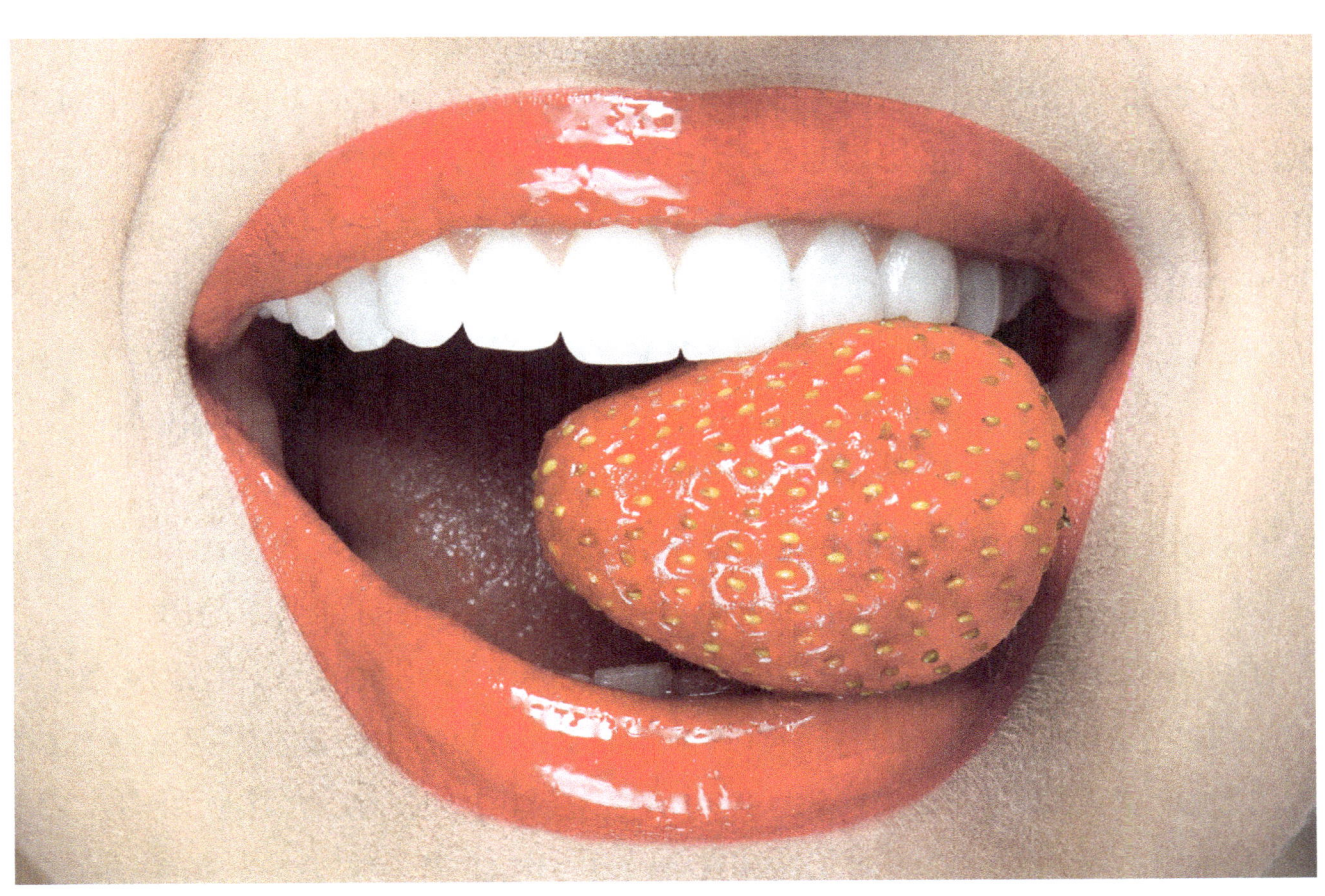

Teeth whitening with strawberries: an effective recipe?

Is it possible to whiten teeth with strawberries? Is this method recommended for whitening? Or is the strawberry whitening recipe unsafe? The answer is in this article.

Teeth whitening with strawberries: an effective recipe?

There are many home and natural teeth whitening recipes, including the strawberry recipe.

Teeth whitening with strawberries: is it an effective recipe?

The use of strawberries may help whiten teeth, and the reason for this is that strawberries contain the following substances:

1. Malic acid

The malic acid content in strawberries may contribute to teeth whitening, as this acid can act as a natural teeth whitening agent.

Malic acid may also help lighten the color of the teeth indirectly due to the ability of this acid to enhance the production of saliva in the mouth, as the presence of sufficient amounts of saliva in the mouth may help to clean the teeth of dirt and food residues, which may contribute to the resistance to tooth decay, which It is one of the common causes of tooth discoloration.

2. Vitamin C and other beneficial substances

It is possible that the benefits and potential effectiveness of the strawberry teeth whitening recipe stem from the fact that strawberries contain vitamin C or the so-called ascorbic acid, in addition to some substances with astringent properties, which together may help remove stains and plaque from the surface of the teeth, which contributes to whitening them. And stimulate it to restore its beautiful natural color.

Other benefits of strawberries for oral health

In addition to strawberries' potential whitening benefits, strawberries may improve oral health in other ways. Strawberries may help prevent periodontal disease or reduce the likelihood of it developing in the mouth.

The benefits of strawberries in this regard may stem from the richness of their delicious berries in vitamin C and antioxidants, which are natural substances that may contribute to strengthening the body's immunity and resistance to infections, which may help inhibit and prevent the growth of harmful oral bacteria that may stimulate the emergence of periodontal disease.

Strawberry teeth whitening methods

Here is a list of the most prominent ways to use strawberries to whiten teeth:

Strawberry and baking soda recipe

One of the popular strawberry teeth whitening recipes is the strawberry recipe with baking soda, and this is how to apply it:

1 Prepare the strawberry baking soda recipe ingredients: 1 strawberry and 1 teaspoon baking soda.
2 Mash the strawberries well, and mix with the fine powdered baking soda.
Put strawberry paste and baking soda on the toothbrush, then brush the teeth.
4 Rinse the teeth with clean water, and re-clean the teeth after that with the brush and paste.
.Repeat the strawberry and baking soda recipe once a week 5

other ways

It is possible to try to whiten teeth with strawberries in other ways, such as the following:

1 chewing gum without sugar and made with strawberries.
2 Apply a small amount of mashed strawberries on the teeth and leave it on the teeth for a few minutes before rinsing the teeth with water.
3 Eat strawberries regularly.

Is strawberry teeth whitening recommended?

The answer is no, as some experts recommend avoiding the use of strawberries for teeth whitening, for the following reasons:

There is some scientific evidence that the use of strawberries has no effect on the color of the teeth, and that it may not help whiten them, contrary to popular belief.

Strawberries contain acids that may have a negative effect on tooth enamel. When strawberries are applied topically on the teeth and left for a while, the acids in strawberries, such as malic acid, may begin to stimulate the dissolution of tooth enamel over time.

It should be noted that this does not mean that you should refrain from eating strawberries, although keeping strawberries on the teeth for a relatively long time may weaken the teeth, but the contact of strawberries with the teeth for a short period while eating may not be harmful.

Other ways to whiten teeth at home

In addition to the strawberry teeth whitening method, these are some other methods that may help to follow once a day to whiten teeth at home and with natural ingredients:

1. Lemon and orange peels

The teeth are rubbed with orange or lemon peels, and the teeth are cleaned after two minutes using the brush and paste before rinsing the mouth with clean water.

2. Coconut oil

Put a spoonful of coconut oil in the mouth, then use this oil to gargle continuously for 10 minutes, after that the oil is spit out and the teeth are cleaned with brush and paste as usual.

3. Apple cider vinegar

Mix two tablespoons or one tablespoon of apple cider vinegar with a cup of water, then use the mixture of vinegar and water as a natural mouthwash, gargling with it for a maximum of 60 seconds, then brushing and toothpaste as usual.

Strawberry Allergy: Your Ultimate Guide

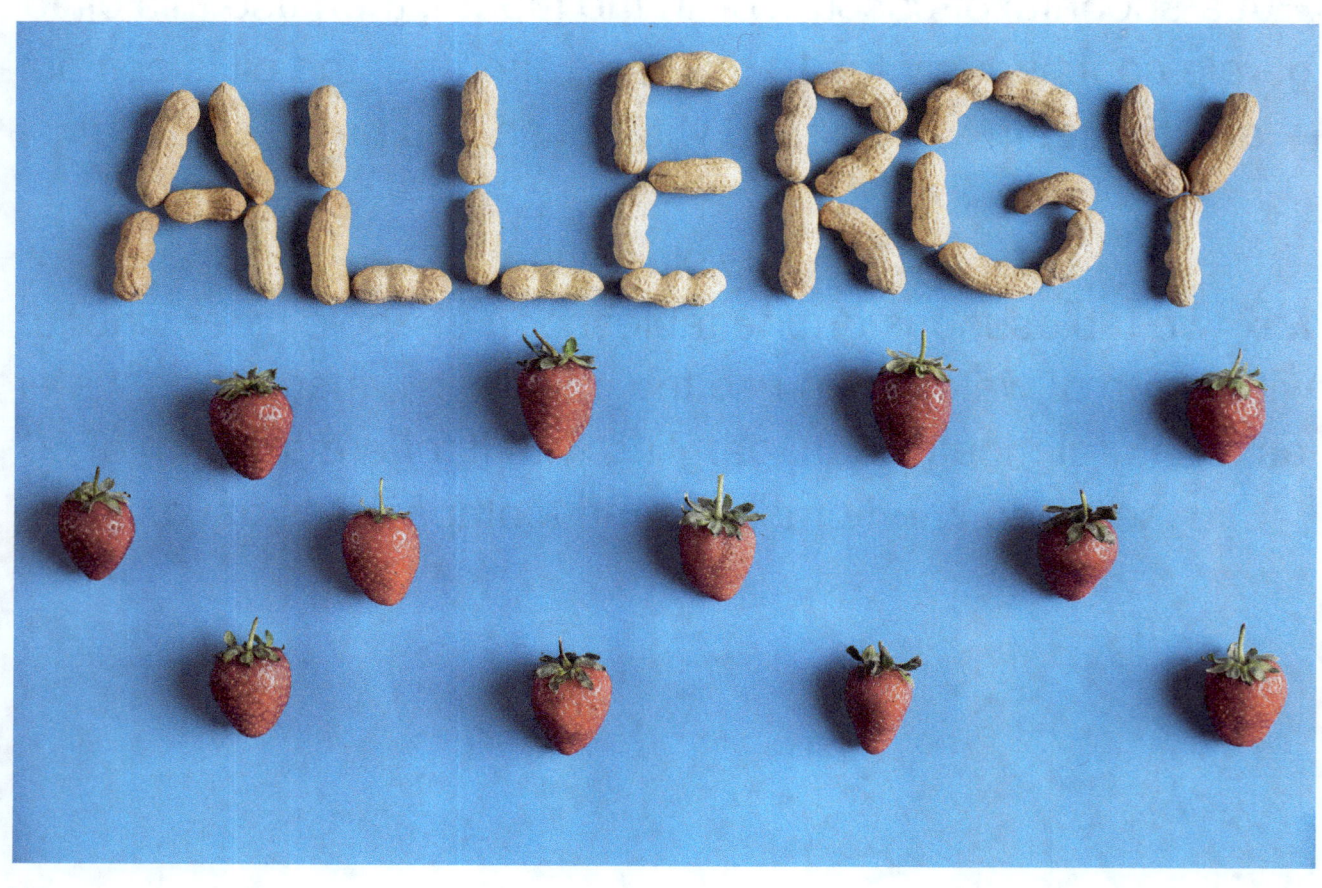

Strawberry Allergy: Your Ultimate Guide

Many people suffer from strawberry allergy when eating them, which leads to the emergence of some painful symptoms, which this article explains.

Strawberry Allergy: Your Ultimate Guide

Strawberries are one of the favorite fruits of many people, but some of them may suffer from strawberry allergy, although it is a less common type of food allergy, and in this case a person may also suffer from an allergy to other fruits of the same family of this plant.

Causes of strawberry allergy

Strawberry allergy is the result of hypersensitivity to the proteins present in strawberries. When they are eaten, the immune system overreacts to these proteins and begins to attack them by forming IgE antibodies.

Antibodies enter the blood and cause the release of histamine from certain cells scattered throughout the body, and histamine causes irritation and inflammation of soft tissues, such as: the sinuses, lungs, and skin.

risk factors

People are more likely to have a food allergy in general and a strawberry allergy in particular if they have the following:

A family history of allergies.

Allergy to birch pollen.

asthma.

Eczema.

Also, young children may be more likely to develop an allergy to a particular food if they are not exposed to it early in their life, as children starting to eat some foods, such as: strawberries at an advanced age, can sometimes lead to an allergic reaction.

Strawberry allergy symptoms

A person with a strawberry allergy is likely to experience only mild to moderate symptoms, which can occur within a few minutes or even a few hours after eating or touching strawberries. The most common symptoms of a strawberry allergy include:

Feeling of tightness in the throat.

Itching or numbness in the mouth.

Skin rash, such as: urticaria or eczema.

itchy skin;

whistling.

cough.

Congestion.

nausea.

stomach pain.

vomiting;

Diarrhea.

;dizziness or lightheadedness

In some cases, strawberry allergy may be severe, leading to a life-threatening allergic reaction called anaphylaxis, which causes many symptoms to occur at the same time and requires emergency medical treatment, and its symptoms include the following:

tongue swelling;
Swelling in the throat blocking the airway.
A sharp drop in blood pressure.
Rapid heartbeat.
dizziness and lightheadedness;
Unconsciousness.
fainting;

strawberry allergy treatment

The best treatment for allergies is to completely avoid the substances that cause them, and in the case of a strawberry allergy, fresh strawberries and their products should be avoided, for example: dried strawberries, strawberry jam, and strawberry candy as well.

In most cases, a person can treat a strawberry allergy at home without medical intervention. Mild or moderate allergies can be treated with antihistamine medications, which do not require a prescription, and they can reduce the severity of symptoms. Severe anaphylaxis need immediate medical attention and should be treated with epinephrine given with a prefilled syringe, so anyone with a known severe allergy needs to have this syringe with them at all times.

Benefits of strawberry for the skin

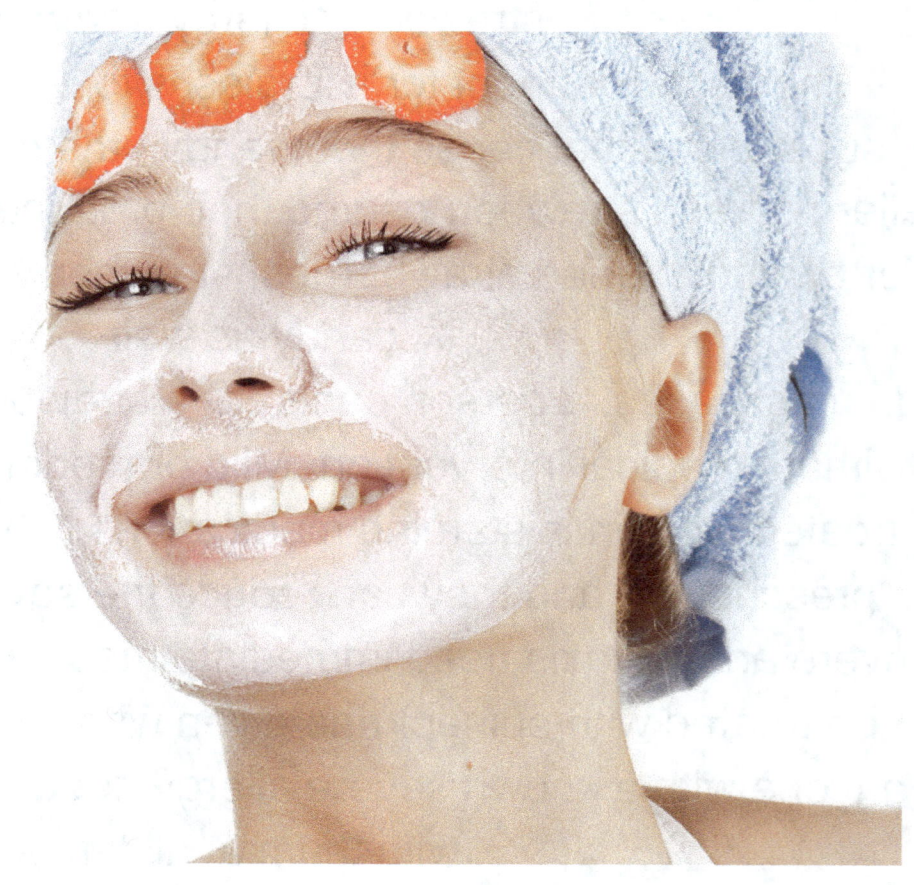

Benefits of strawberry for the skin

What are the main benefits of strawberry for the skin? How can these benefits be obtained? Learn all of that and more through this article.

Benefits of strawberry for the skin

Strawberries include many natural elements that may dispense with the use of regular cosmetic products, and here are some of the benefits of strawberries for the skin:

Benefits of strawberry for the skin

Here is a list of the most prominent benefits of strawberries for the skin:

fight aging

Strawberries contain an acid known as ellagic acid that fights UV damage by blocking enzymes from destroying collagen, preventing wrinkles and making the skin look healthy and radiant.

Prevent acne breakouts

Strawberries may help get rid of the sebum accumulated in the pores of the skin that causes acne, as it is one of the citrus fruits that enhances its properties.

Protects the skin from skin cancer

As mentioned earlier, strawberries contain ellagic acid, which protects the skin from harmful sunlight, and this not only helps reduce wrinkles, but may protect the skin from skin cancer.

Contributes to skin lightening

Strawberries can be effective in lightening skin tone and getting rid of acne scars, thanks to ellagic acid and other active ingredients that contribute to it.

Reduces dark circles and wrinkles around the eyes

Strawberries contain an excellent percentage of vitamin C, which promotes collagen production in the skin, which contributes to reducing the appearance of wrinkles and fine lines around the eyes, and the omega-3 fatty acids in it help lighten the area around the eyes and remove dark circles.

Improve skin health

Alpha hydroxy acids (Alpha hydroxy) present in strawberries help rid the skin of dead skin cells and cleanse it deeply, and it also treats the problem of dullness and roughness of the skin. Strawberries also contain salicylic acid, which can help reduce hyperpigmentation and dark spots, and is even used in skin care products designed to remove dead skin cells, tighten pores, and cleanse the skin of bacteria and dirt, which contributes to significantly reducing the appearance of pimples. .
Moreover, Vitamin C helps calm irritated skin and boost its vitality.

How to get the benefits of strawberry for the skin

In addition to eating strawberries, they can be used in the following ways:

1. Strawberry and honey mask

In addition to strawberries, honey is known for its moisturizing and emollient properties for the skin. This mask is especially useful for fighting blemishes and acne. It is prepared as follows:

Ingredients
It includes:

3 pieces of fresh strawberries.
1 tablespoon of honey.

How to prepare and use
The following steps are followed:

1 Mash the strawberries until smooth, then add the honey and stir together.
2 Apply the mixture to clean skin using a sterile brush or clean fingers, avoiding the eye area.
3 Leave the mask on the skin for 15 minutes, then wash it off with warm water and apply the appropriate toner and moisturizer for the skin.

2. Strawberry Scrub

As mentioned earlier, strawberries contain alpha hydroxy acids that exfoliate the skin, and can be used as follows:

Ingredients
It includes fresh strawberries as needed only.

How to prepare and use
The following steps are followed:

1 cut strawberry into slices.
2 Scrub the entire face and eye area with strawberry slices for a few minutes.
.Wash the face well and moisturize it 3

Benefits of strawberry for the skin

Oral consumption of strawberries is safe for most people if this consumption is within the normal limits far from excessive, but it may cause allergic reactions in some, and this also applies to its application on the skin, and its most prominent damages include the following:

Skin allergy.
Irritability and redness of the skin.
blisters appear
itching;
Increased risk of bleeding and bruising in people with bleeding disorders.
Slowing blood clotting and increasing the risk of bleeding during and after surgery.

strawberry mask recipes

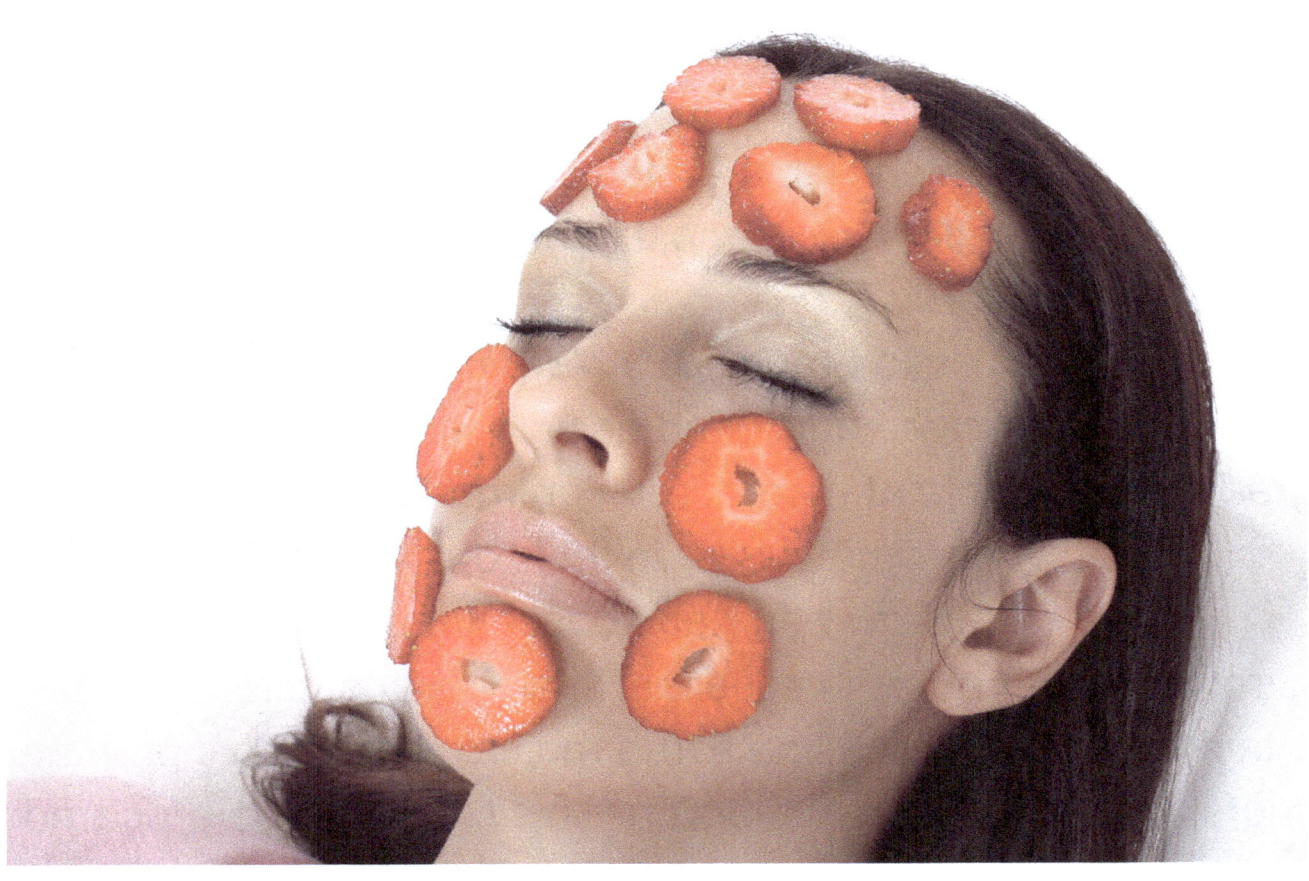

strawberry mask recipes

Want to naturally boost your skin's health? We offer you many recipes for the perfect strawberry mask to take care of your beauty.

strawberry mask recipes

Even if your skin is fresh and healthy, there must come a day when you look tired and pale. The best thing you can do to boost your skin and reduce the chance of dullness is to provide it with water, vitamin C, and antioxidants, and strawberries are one of the fruits rich in skin enhancers.

So let's get acquainted with the methods of preparing a strawberry mask for the face, and its most important benefits as follows:

How to prepare a strawberry mask

You can make these quick and easy to make face masks with ingredients available at home. You can make them in five minutes every time your skin feels dull and dry:

Strawberry and cocoa mask

Strawberries are rich in essential vitamins and minerals. They contain vitamin C, which fights free radicals and delays premature aging. It also helps lighten the skin. This mask can be prepared as follows:

1. Ingredients
Bring the following components:
- 4 pieces of strawberry.
- A tablespoon of cocoa powder.
- A teaspoon of honey.

2. Method of preparation
Follow these steps to prepare this mask:
- Blend the strawberries in a blender until they become a paste, then put them in a bowl.
- Add cocoa powder and honey to the strawberries.
- Apply the mask to your face, leave it for 15 minutes, and then wash it off with warm water.

Strawberry and aloe vera mask
Here is how to prepare a mask of strawberry and aloe vera gel that is beneficial for your skin:

1. Ingredients
Prepare the following ingredients:
- A large strawberry.
- A tablespoon of aloe vera gel.
- Dry milk as needed.

2. Method of preparation
All you have to do to prepare this mask is the following:
1. Mash the strawberries well and try to get rid of all lumps.
2. Mix the strawberries with the aloe vera gel.
3. Add enough dry milk to get a smooth paste that is neither too thick nor too loose.
4. Apply the mask on your face after cleaning it, and leave it for 20 minutes.
5. Wash your face using lukewarm water, then apply the appropriate face cream for your skin type

Strawberry and banana mask

Strawberry and banana mask helps remove skin blemishes, and reduce the chance of their appearance.

To prepare this mask, all you have to do is:

1 Mash 1/4 cup of bananas, along with 1/4 cup of strawberries.
2 Add 1/4 cup of sour cream or yogurt, and 1 tablespoon of honey to the mixture.
3 Apply it on your face for a quarter of an hour before washing it with warm water.

Benefits of strawberry mask for the skin

The benefits of strawberry mask for the skin include all of the following:

Strawberries contain ellagic acid, which works to protect the skin from UV damage by blocking enzymes that contribute to the destruction of collagen, and this helps prevent wrinkles from forming on the skin.

The high amount of Vitamin C present in strawberries helps in lightening the skin.

The astringent properties in addition to the antioxidants present in strawberries contribute to the treatment of puffiness in the eye area, and reduce inflammation in the skin.

Strawberries are rich in alpha hydroxy acid, which gets rid of dead skin cells, and salicylic acid, which is ideal for treating acne.

Manganese and antioxidants both tone the skin.

Strawberry mask side effects

Some people may have a strawberry allergy, which can cause rashes and skin infections.

Therefore, it is recommended to test a small amount of the strawberry mask on a small area of your skin before continuing to apply it completely.

Meet the white strawberry

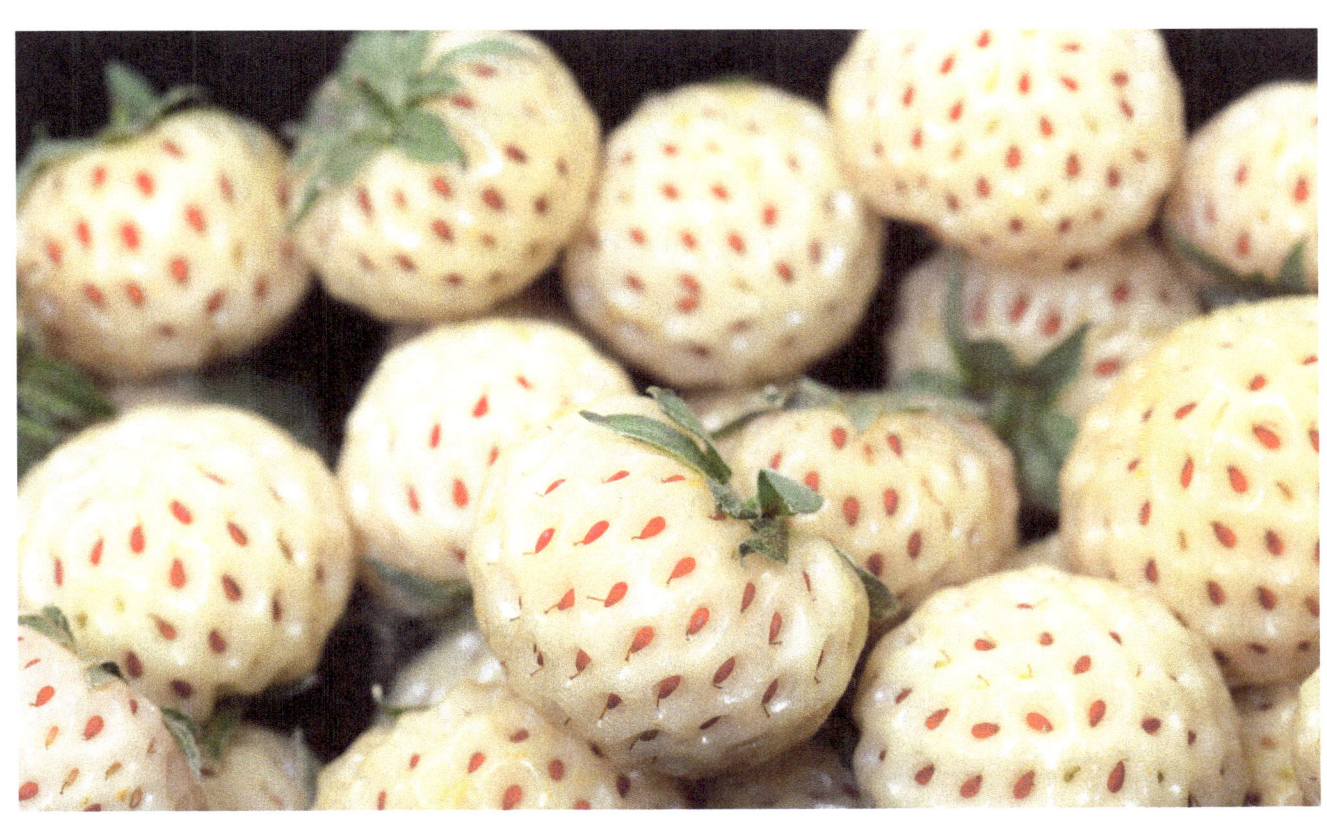

Meet the white strawberry

What is white strawberry? And what is the benefit? What is the difference between it and the red strawberry?

Meet the white strawberry

Red strawberries spread in the Middle East, but what are white strawberries? Here is the answer.

white strawberry

The white strawberry is one of the uncommon and rare fruits in general.

Since red strawberries are the most common in the region, and white strawberries grow naturally in Europe and South America, white strawberries are classified into two types according to where they grow, namely:

- Alpine strawberry (Fragaria vesca), which is the most popular.
- Beach strawberry (Fragaria chiloensis).

The beach strawberry has been crossed to give it a white color and a sweeter taste.

What is the difference between white and red strawberries?

To answer the question, it is necessary to know the life cycle of strawberries, which is explained by the following:

- The flowers turn into small green strawberries the size of a pea.
- Small green strawberries grow to a certain size and ripen, then turn white.

As they continue to ripen, strawberries that are red when fully ripe benefit from the proteins to turn from white to red.
As for white strawberries, they are deficient or completely lacking in this protein so even when ripe they stay white instead of turning red.

The genes for strawberries do not allow them to become red, so the reason white strawberries are white is simply because they lack the ability to turn red.

white strawberry cultivation

White strawberries are perennial plants that are easy to grow either in the garden or in containers, and strawberries can be grown in the home garden, by following these steps:

Choose a suitable area that receives sunlight 6 hours a day, and is protected from cold and frost.
Choose clay soil and fertilize it with organic matter before planting.
Planting seeds or seedlings so that the distance between each seedling is 30 centimeters.
Planting in spring or fall when the outside temperature is around 15°C.
Plant the seedlings until the soil completely covers the roots, so that the crown is on the surface of the soil.
Maintain constant irrigation and use drip irrigation.
The strawberries will be ready for harvest (4-6) weeks after planting.
Strawberries are stored in a closed container in the refrigerator for a week.

white strawberry price

The white strawberry has a higher price when compared to the traditional red strawberry, as it is considered one of the luxury fruits in the Japanese market. The reason for the high price of white strawberry is due to:

Because of the years it takes strawberries to reproduce.
Its low production rate.
The process of growing and growing it is expensive.
Although strawberries are not huge in size, you need to allocate a lot of space to grow properly.

strawberry allergy

Some people have an allergy to strawberries, and this allergy comes from the protein (Fragariaergen A1), which gives strawberries their red color.

Which results in some allergic reaction, when eating red strawberries.

Individuals with strawberry allergy are advised to consume white strawberries, to avoid negative side effects or allergic reactions.

Health benefits of strawberries

There are a number of benefits that accrue to the body with health and benefit, and among these benefits are the following:

Circulatory system protection: by reducing the risk of heart disease, preventing high cholesterol, and raising good fats in the body.

Control blood pressure: by reducing sudden high blood pressure.

Rich in nutrients: strawberries are a good source of fiber, proteins, minerals and vitamins, which are necessary to carry out vital functions.

Strengthen the immune system: Strawberries contain polyphenols, an antioxidant that works to boost immunity.

Learn about the benefits of strawberries for men

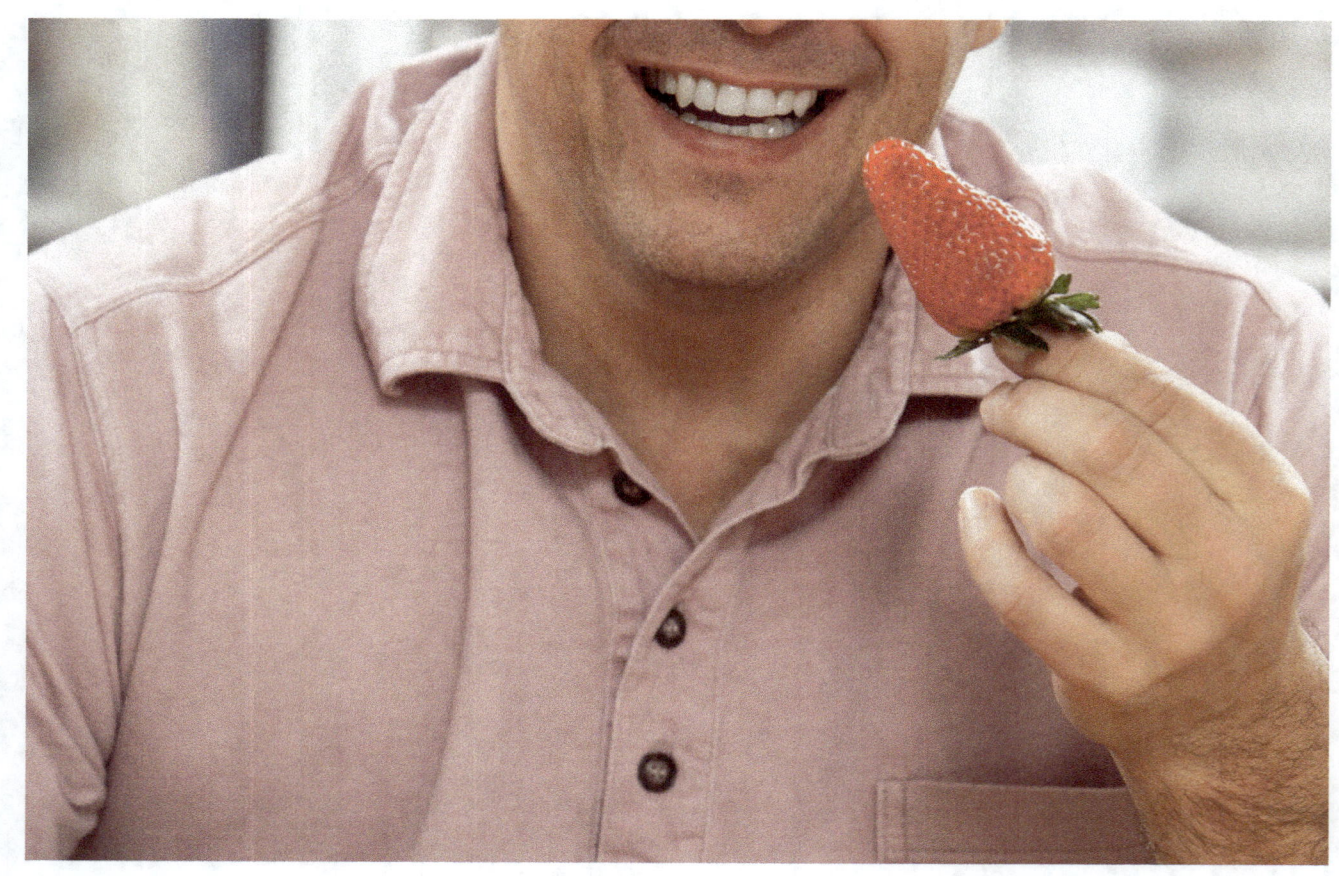

Learn about the benefits of strawberries for men

What do you know about the benefits of strawberries for men? Are there other foods that may be useful for men? Find out the answer through this article.

Learn about the benefits of strawberries for men

Have you ever thought about the benefits of strawberries for men? In this article we will answer your questions on this topic:

What are the benefits of strawberry for men?

The benefits of strawberry for men are numerous, but of course there is a need for more research to confirm this, which is summarized in the following points:

1. Increase testosterone

Strawberries contain zinc, which may help increase testosterone production, which is responsible for sperm production.

Its deficiency leads to fertility problems, so strawberries are important for men.

2. Increased blood flow

Strawberries are rich in antioxidants that help increase blood flow to the reproductive organs, which contributes to supporting and maintaining a man's sexual health.

3. Erection

Strawberries contain vitamin C, which may help increase sexual desire in men, and it also helps prevent prostate problems that may help impede erection.

4. Power supply

Strawberries help provide you with energy, which is essential in intercourse, and in addition, they have a low glycemic index, so you can eat them to provide you with energy without thinking about calories.

What are the other benefits of strawberries?

After we have finished talking about the most prominent benefits of strawberries for men, we will move on to talking about the benefits of strawberries for men and women, or their benefits in general, including the following:

1. Helps prevent heart disease

Strawberries contain many compounds that help prevent heart disease, such as:

Natural anti-inflammatory compounds may help prevent atherosclerosis.

Polyphenol compound.

potassium and fibre.

2. Contribute to the prevention of clots

Strawberries are rich in antibiotics that may help prevent strokes, but more research is needed to confirm this.

It is worth noting that adding strawberries to the diet is a good and healthy addition, however, it should be eaten in moderation.

3. It is believed to have a role in preventing cancer

Some foods, such as strawberries, help prevent cancer because they contain antioxidants, but it is not possible to say for sure, and there is a need for more research to support the validity of this statement.

4. Contribute to lowering blood pressure

Strawberries contain high amounts of potassium, which may help lower blood pressure, and research indicates that the risk of not eating potassium in affecting blood pressure is equal to the risk of eating too much sodium, so strawberries are a good way to provide potassium to the body.

5. Regulate blood sugar

Strawberries help regulate blood sugar, due to their high fiber content, in addition, fiber increases satiety, and thus will reduce the amount of meals that contain sugar.

Are there other foods useful for men?

After we finish talking about the benefits of strawberries for men and their benefits in general, we will move on to talking about some other natural foods that may be useful for them, including the following:

1 Spinach: Spinach may help increase blood flow towards the penis, due to its folic acid content, which helps with an erection.
2. Apples: Apples can help prevent prostate diseases, but more research is needed to confirm this.
3 Avocados: Avocados may help increase fertility, as they contain vitamin E, which in turn may help improve sperm quality. And Carrots: Carrots can help increase sperm count and motility, but 4 more research is needed to confirm this.

The benefits of strawberries for women: fact or myth?

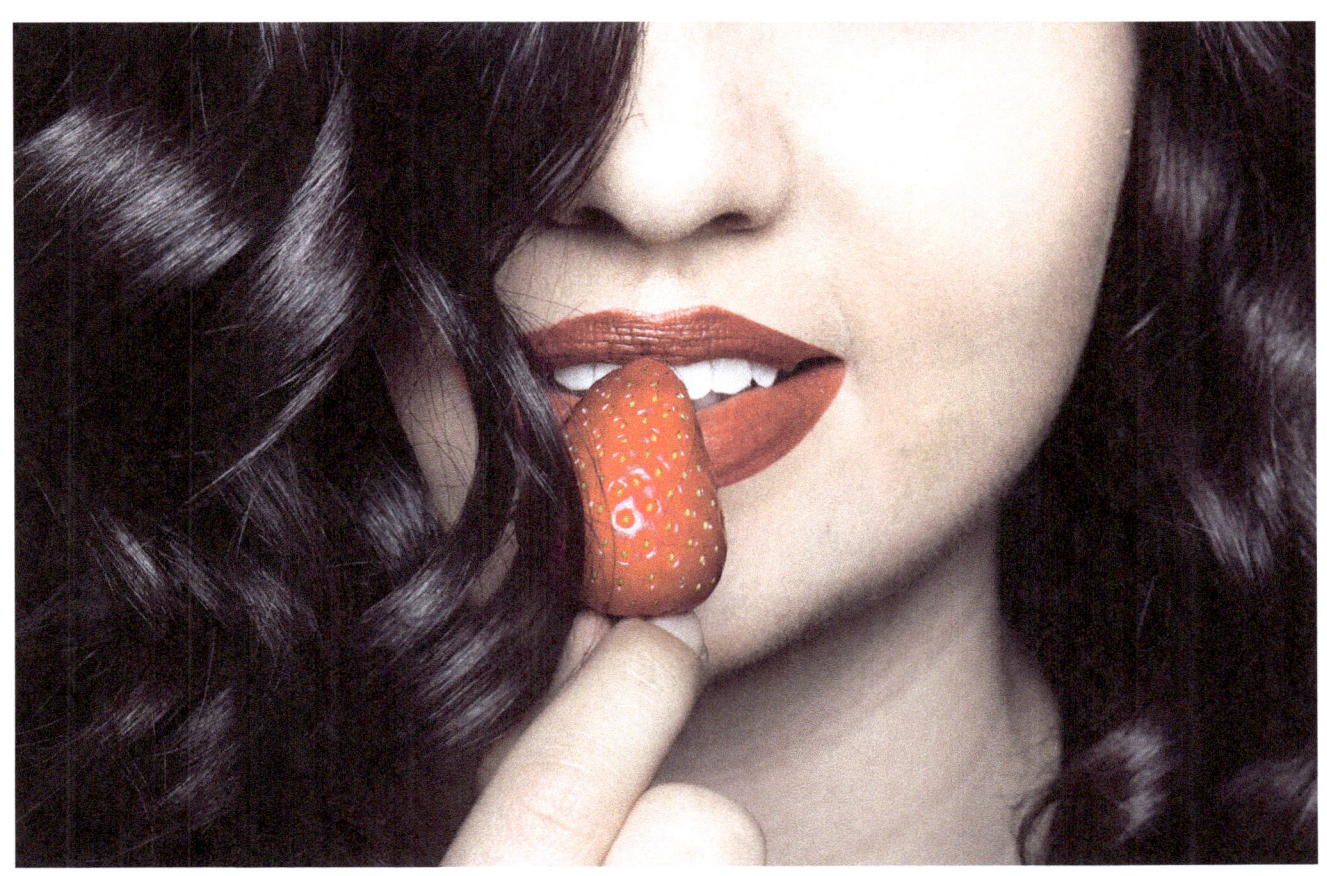

The benefits of strawberries for women: fact or myth?

The benefits of strawberries for women: fact or myth?

In the following, we will learn about the benefits of strawberries for women:

strawberry benefits for women

There are many benefits that strawberries provide only for women, here are the most prominent in the following:

1. Reducing menstruation symptoms

During menstruation, women often feel unpleasant symptoms, such as: an urgent desire to eat sweets, which may cause them health problems later, some foods may contribute to alleviating these symptoms.

Eating sweet-tasting strawberries during menstruation may help satisfy a woman's desire for sugar without raising the level of glucose in the blood above the normal limit, which in turn reduces the incidence of diabetes and obesity.

2. Preventing the fetus from having birth defects

A pregnant woman's getting enough folic acid is essential to keep the fetus healthy from the risks of pregnancy.

Folic acid helps prevent birth defects in the fetus, especially the brain. Failure to obtain the recommended amounts from the doctor may cause the child after birth to develop a defect in the brain and spinal cord, which in turn leads to anencephaly and spina bifida in the spine. (Spina bifida).

Strawberries are rich in folic acid with 10% of the recommended daily intake for pregnant women.

3. Breast cancer prevention

Strawberries contain ellagic acid, an anti-cancer plant chemical that slows down the progression of cancer cells and destroys types of them, and can reduce the risk of breast, skin, lung and bladder cancers.

Strawberries are also a fruit rich in fiber and vitamin C, which both contribute to protecting the body from esophageal and colon cancer.

Benefits of strawberry for women and men

Strawberries have many benefits, the benefits of strawberries for women and men alike are as follows:

Controls blood sugar: Strawberries are low in sugar in addition to fiber, which prevents blood sugar levels from rising above the normal limit.

Strengthens the bones: Strawberries reduce the risk of worsening symptoms of osteoarthritis in the knee, and prevent them from developing inflammation.

Strengthens the body's immunity: Strawberries are one of the foods rich in vitamin C, which strengthens the immune system, especially during the winter season, when the risk of influenza is high.

Helps in weight loss: The high levels of fiber in strawberries contribute to controlling cravings, and the number of calories in this fruit is low.

Skin cell renewal: Salicylic acid present in strawberries helps get rid of dead skin cells, giving the skin its freshness, and tightens pores, which prevents acne.

Teeth whitening: Strawberries contain malic acid, which removes pigmentation from the teeth.

Tips for women eating strawberries

After you know the benefits of strawberries for women, here are the most important tips that will boost your health:

Eat strawberries in moderation, as you should not eat more than eight strawberries per day.

Make sure to wash and scrub the strawberries well with water and then dry them before eating them.

Avoid over-applying strawberries on the teeth, as this may erode the enamel layer.

Add strawberries to your food dishes if you do not prefer to eat them alone, you can drink it as a juice or mix it with salad or cake.

Make sure that you are not allergic to strawberries before eating them. Go to the doctor in case you get dizzy, short of breath, or have a rash after eating them.

Benefits of strawberry for pregnant women

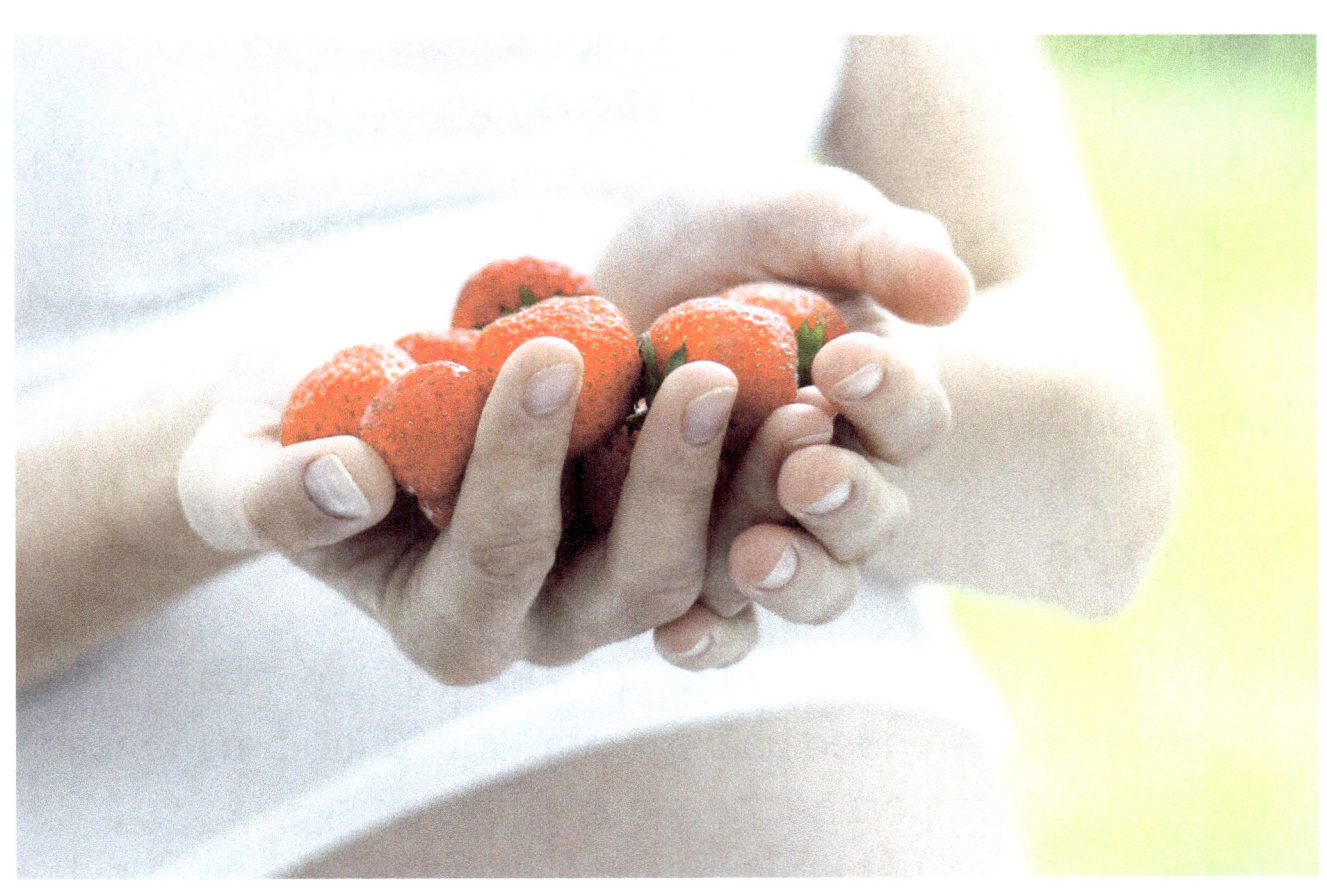

Benefits of strawberry for pregnant women

Strawberries are delicious fruits and very rich in vitamins, but what are the benefits of strawberries for pregnant women?

Benefits of strawberry for pregnant women

You should know that the benefits of strawberry for pregnant women are numerous, so a pregnant woman should include it in her diet and should not avoid eating it at all.

Benefits of strawberry for pregnant women

Here are the most important benefits of strawberries for pregnant women in the following:

Very rich in vitamin C, as one cup of strawberries provides the nutritional need of the pregnant woman, which is important in raising the efficiency of the immune system of the pregnant woman and is very necessary to build collagen, which is important in building your child's bones and cartilage.

They contain a large amount of ellagic acid which is very important for the gut health of you and your baby.

It contains 7% of the folic acid a pregnant woman needs, which in turn prevents birth defects in your child's spinal cord.

Rich in substances that help reduce harmful cholesterol in the body and plaque in the arteries.

The vitamin A present in it helps to strengthen eyesight and protect the retina of the eye.

Reducing the chance of anemia, because it is very rich in iron, as a pregnant woman needs a large amount during pregnancy to support her health and her fetus.

It is very rich in fiber that helps prevent constipation during pregnancy.

Strawberries are low in calories and can be eaten as snacks during the day.

strawberry nutritional value

For the nutritional value and available elements of one cup of strawberries see the following table:

nutritional element	Available value
Energy	50 calories
Carbohydrates	12 grams
Fiber	1.96 g
Calcium	19.6 milligrams
Iron	0.71 milligrams
Vitamin A	0 IU
Vitamin C	60.1 milligrams

Tips for eating strawberries during pregnancy

Some tips when eating strawberries to get all the benefits of strawberries for pregnant women are as follows:

It is advised to avoid eating strawberries if you have a family history of strawberry allergy, even if you do not have strawberry allergy symptoms.

Wash strawberries well before eating them to remove bacteria and parasites such as E. coli from the soil and get rid of dirt and fertilizer residues.

Do not rely on strawberries alone for the full portion of fruits and make them part of the daily portion to get a variety of vitamins and minerals.

Choose fresh or frozen whole strawberries and stay away from jams or strawberry flavors because they contain more sugar and less fiber.

If you want to get strawberries in juice form, make sure that the prepared juice is pasteurized to avoid the risk of bacterial infection.

Ways to include strawberries in the diet

A group of ways to help you increase the consumption of strawberries to get more benefits of strawberries for the pregnant woman, including:

Add strawberries with Greek yogurt and fresh juices.
Put it on toast instead of jam.
Add it to your morning breakfast cereal.
Prepare a salad and mix it with more fruits.
Use strawberries as a garnish for cakes and pies.
Dip it in dark chocolate rich in antioxidants.
.Freeze it to enjoy it all year round

strawberry for babies

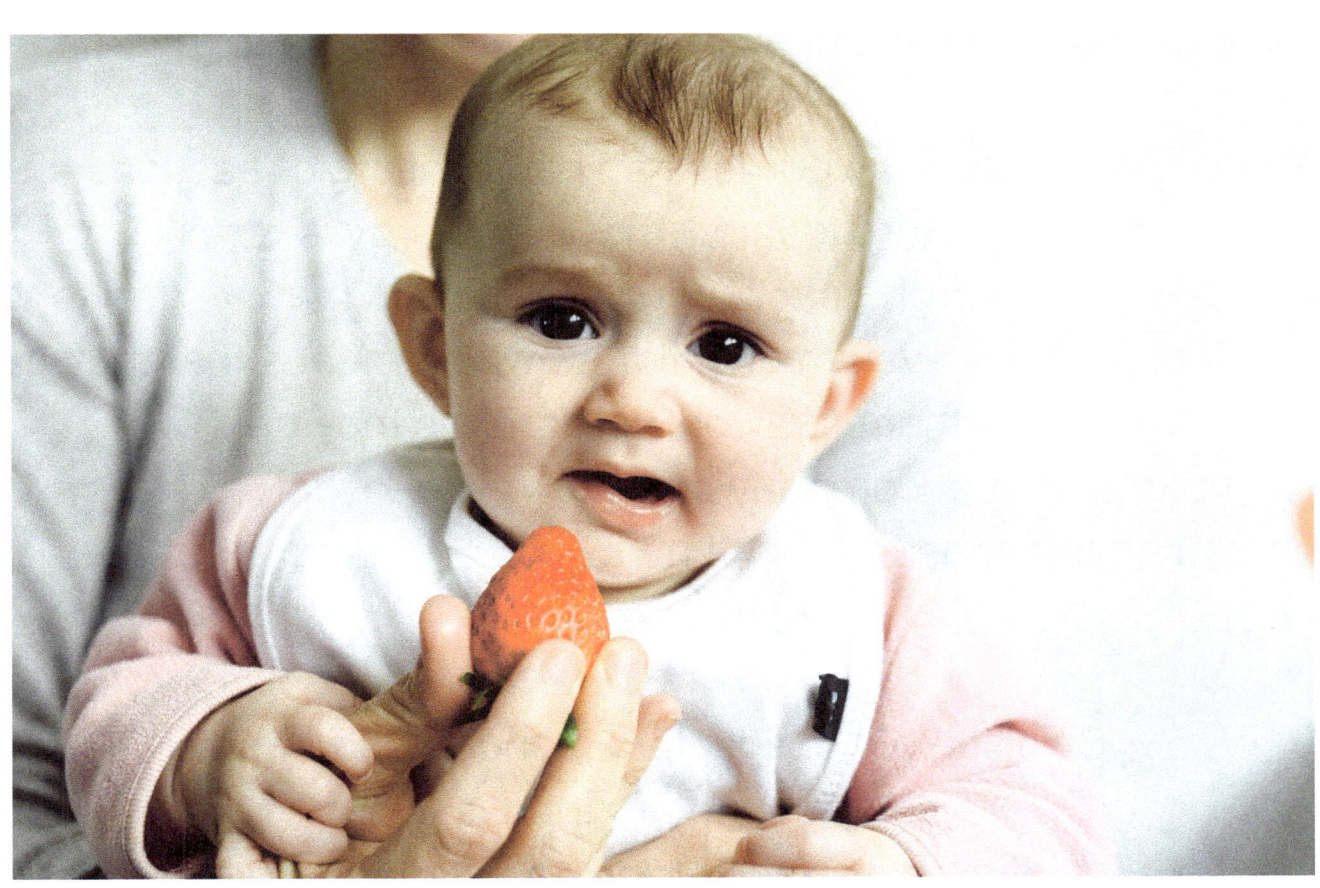

strawberry for babies

What distinguishes strawberries is their wonderful nutritional value, as they are rich in vitamin C and B and other vitamins and minerals, but what should you know about strawberries for infants?

strawberry for babies

When can strawberries be given to infants, what are their health benefits, and how can they be presented to a child? The answers are in this article.

When can strawberries be fed to infants?

It is preferable to introduce strawberries to infants after about 12 months, or after they have learned how to chew food, because they can cause choking if given to them in the form of a large fruit.

strawberry allergy

On the other hand, strawberries can cause allergic reactions, but it is important to know that this allergy is rare.

Sometimes an allergic reaction to strawberries may be due to the immature immune system of children, which means that they can try to feed them strawberries later as they get older.

Symptoms that accompany strawberry allergy for infants vary according to exposure to it. If he touches it, he may suffer from these symptoms:

- rash
- Swelling of the lips, face, tongue and throat
- Tongue numbness

In the case of eating strawberries, the symptoms include the following:

- Nausea and vomiting
- stomach cramps;
- diarrhea

1. Strawberry gentlemen

Ingredients:

5 pieces of strawberry.

a glass of water.

The way it works:

1 Wash the strawberries well with water and a little apple cider vinegar to get rid of bacteria, then dry them and cut them into quarters.

2 If the strawberries are separated, steam them for three minutes, then rinse them using cold water and leave them in a colander for three minutes to cool.

3 Puree the strawberries in a blender until smooth, then add water as needed to reach the desired consistency.

Note: Leftovers can be stored in the freezer for up to three months.

2. Strawberry and Banana

Ingredients:

A cup of sliced banana.

A cup of sliced strawberries.

Three or four glasses of water or milk.

The way it works:

1 Mash the bananas, you can use a fork because they are soft. Add the banana to the strawberry in the electric mixer, and it is 2 possible to add water and milk to get the desired consistency and suitable for your child.

The benefits of strawberry for children here are the most important

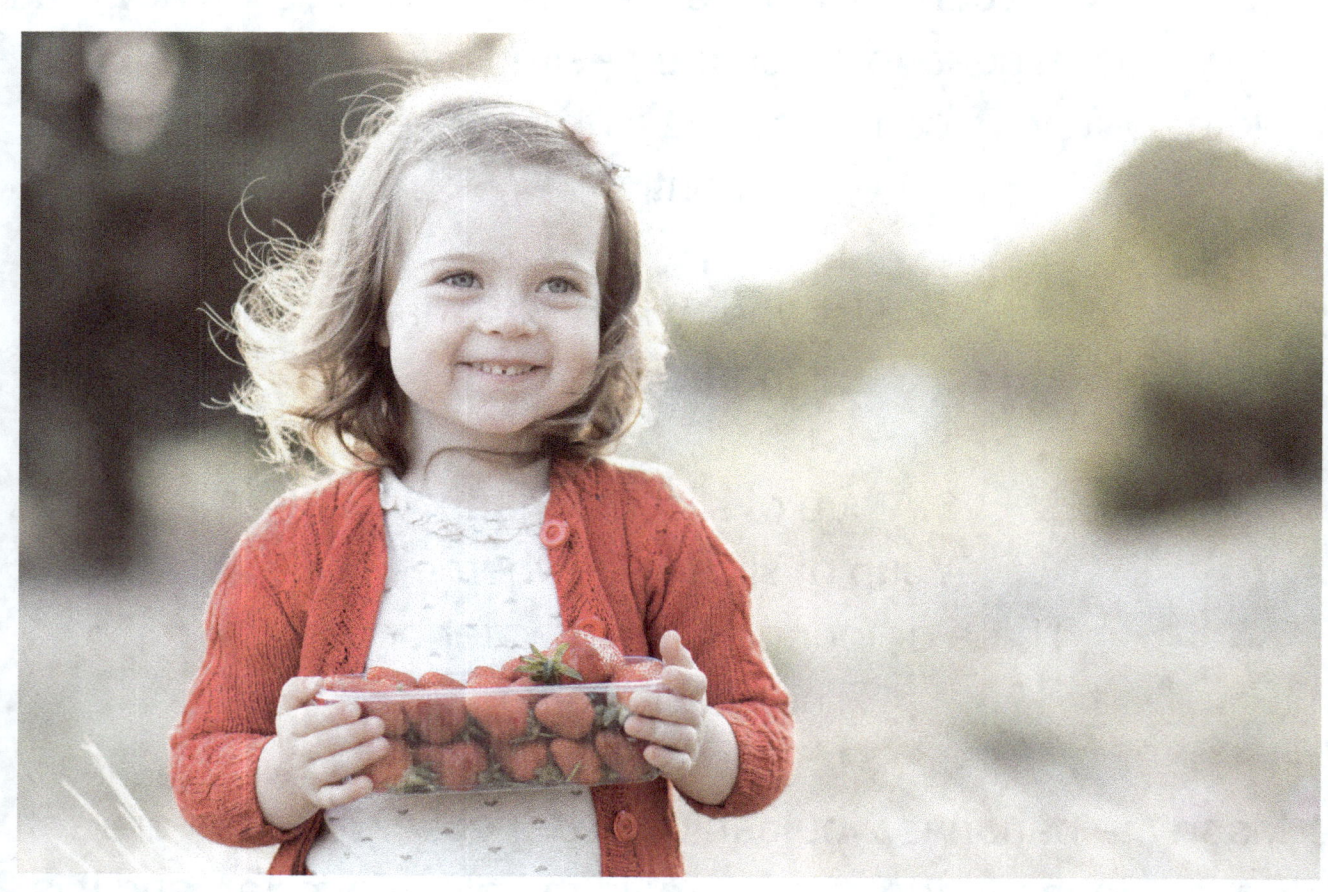

The benefits of strawberries for children: here are the most important ones

Strawberries have many benefits for children's health, as they contain a lot of nutrients. Learn about the benefits of strawberries for children.

The benefits of strawberries for children: here are the most important ones

Although strawberries are one of the most popular fruits in the world, they are loved by children and youngsters, and have many benefits, but care must be taken before feeding them to children, as they may cause an allergic reaction.

Doctors usually recommend avoiding giving strawberries to children under one year, especially those whose parents are allergic to strawberries.

Let's get acquainted with the benefits of strawberries for children and their importance:

strawberry benefits for kids

We offer you the benefits of strawberry for children, which are as follows:

1. Nourishing for children

Strawberry is a fruit rich in many nutrients, which makes it among the most important benefits of strawberries for children.

They contain vitamins, fiber, and high levels of antioxidants known as polyphenols, which are essential for your child's health.

Strawberries are also on the list of foods free of sodium, cholesterol, and calories.

They are ranked among the best fruits for antioxidants, and they are also a good source of manganese and potassium. Eight strawberries contain more vitamin C than an orange.

2. Immune booster

Vitamin C must be obtained from external sources as your child's body cannot process it on its own.

Strawberries are a good source of vitamin C that helps your child build his immunity and prevent eye diseases.

3. Essential for bones

Calcium is one of the necessary things that you must provide for your child. It helps in the growth of bones and improves the work of the heart, muscles and nerves of the child. Among the benefits of strawberries for children is that it is a rich source of calcium.

4. Useful for digestion

The phosphorous in strawberries can improve your child's digestion, aid in cell repair, and break down protein responsible for regulating chemical reactions that occur in your child's body.

5. Protects the liver

Strawberries are a fruit rich in antioxidants, which can reduce oxidative stress and prevent liver damage.

6. Promotes Brain Health

Strawberries are rich in folic acid, which is essential for your baby's brain development, and also helps in the production of red blood cells.

7. Useful for diabetics

Strawberries are a healthy fruit choice for children with diabetes, as their fiber content helps in regulating the blood sugar level, and keeps it stable by avoiding high and low levels.

Fiber can keep your child feeling full long after eating, which reduces the desire to snack between meals, which supports glucose management and reduces the risk of high blood sugar.

Strawberry juice recipe for kids

To get the benefits of strawberry for children, include his daily meals in moderate quantities, we offer you a healthy and nutritious strawberry juice recipe for your child.

Ingredients:
1 cup of unsweetened pineapple chunks.
2 and a half cups of chopped strawberries.
3 teaspoons of honey.
4 cups of low-fat soy milk.
5 ½ cup of yogurt.

How to prepare:
1 Place the pineapple pieces and strawberries in a blender.
2 Add soy milk, honey and yogurt.
3 Serve it to your child after you get a smooth consistency of strawberry juice.

You should also make sure that your child is not allergic to strawberries before serving them.

What are the signs of strawberry allergy in infants?

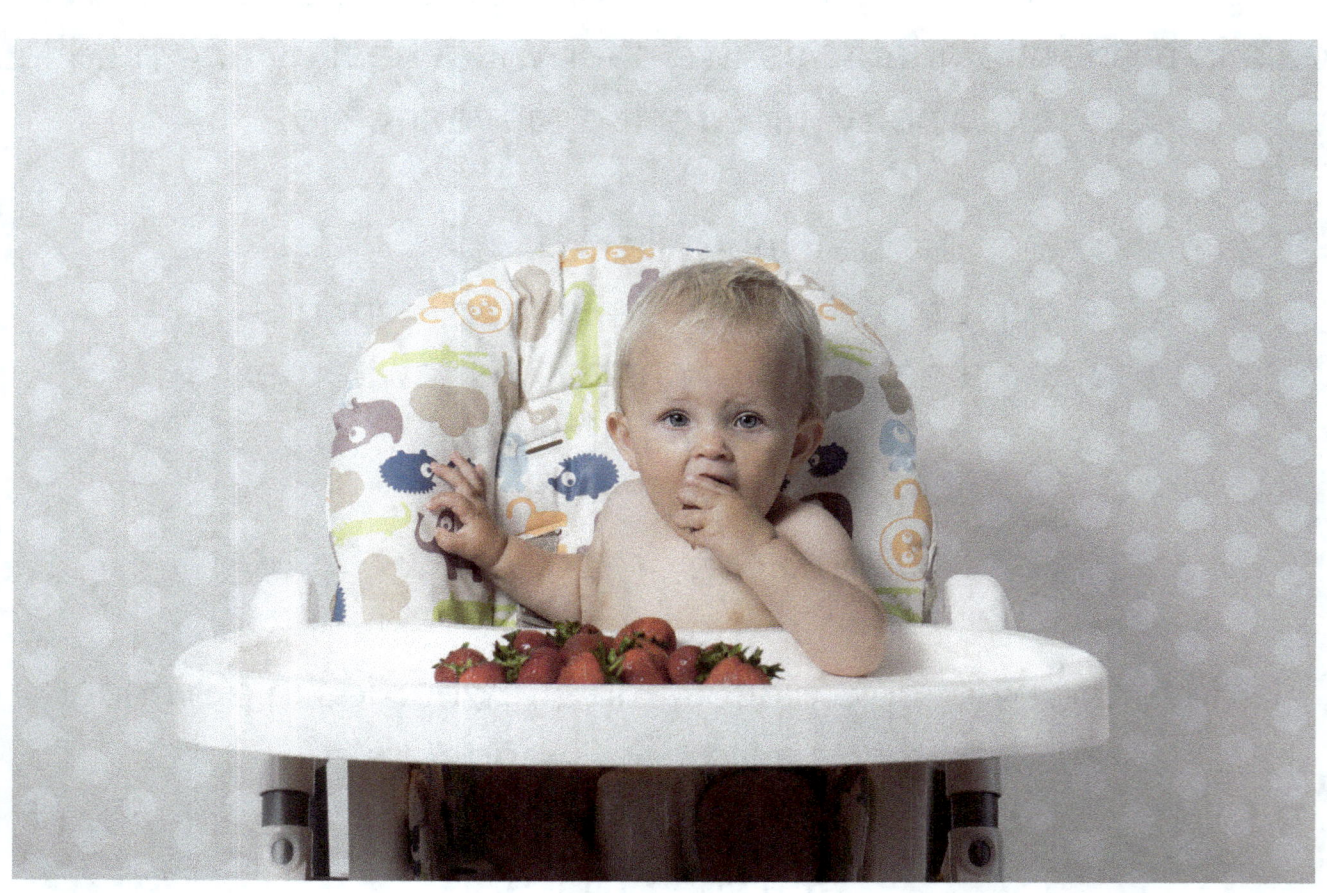

What are the signs of strawberry allergy in infants?

Food allergy is common in infants, and strawberry allergy falls under it. What are the symptoms of strawberry allergy in infants? Details in the following article.

What are the signs of strawberry allergy in infants?

When a child with a strawberry allergy is exposed to strawberries, whether by touching, eating or even smelling them, the immune system is stimulated against it, producing antibodies and stimulating mast cells to produce a substance called histamine, which causes many symptoms, in the following article many details about strawberry allergy in infants:

What are the indications of strawberry allergy in infants?

Evidence of strawberry allergy in infants is divided into two parts, as follows:

1. Mild to moderate signs

The appearance of these symptoms requires a doctor's visit to make sure that the allergy is caused by eating strawberries:

- Itching and rash
- Eczema
- Swelling of the face, eyes, or mouth as a result of angioedema
- Tingling or numbness in the throat and around the mouth
- dry cough
- Congestion, runny nose and sneezing
- Vomiting and colic
- Loose stools
- Baby's mood changes, including constant crying
- Slurred speech if the child is already speaking
- The child pulled his ears
- Unusually, the child pulled his tongue and placed the hand over the mouth.

2. Severe clues

It means anaphylactic shock, which poses a threat to the life of the infant and therefore requires urgent medical intervention. Symptoms of this condition include the following:

Rapid heartbeat.
Breathing difficulty.
Enlargement of the larynx and tongue.
Hearing a whistling sound from the airways when the infant breathes.
Dizziness or fainting.
Reduction of Blood pressure.

How does strawberry allergy occur in infants?
Strawberry allergy occurs in infants when a child with an allergy to strawberries is exposed to strawberries, whether by eating, touching, or smelling.

Risk factors that increase the chance of developing a strawberry allergy in infants
The following groups are most susceptible to strawberry allergy:

Asthma patients.
Eczema sufferers.
Children with a family history of a similar illness, such as a family member having a strawberry allergy.
.People with pollen allergy

Recommendations when serving strawberries to babies

Experts recommend exposing infants to foods that are likely to cause an allergy before their first birthday, with 2015 research supporting the idea that exposing a child to food early can significantly reduce the chance of an allergy later.

Here are recommendations to ensure that strawberries are served to babies without complications:

1 Rub a very small amount of strawberries on the child's lips to notice any signs of allergy and wait a few hours, in the event that no symptoms appear, add a small amount equivalent to a quarter of a mashed spoon, for example, to the child's normal food, mix it well and present it to the child and then monitor any changes, if nothing happens, the quantity can be increased Gradually monitor any changes that may occur with the child.

2 Not to expose the child's skin to strawberries, as it does not help at all in determining whether the child is allergic or not, but it may be a trigger for the occurrence of strawberry allergy with the infant later.

3 If there is a history of strawberry allergy in a family member, please consult a specialized pediatrician, who will often advise exposing the child to strawberries for the first time under medical supervision.

What should I do if my child has a strawberry allergy?

Unfortunately, there is not yet a medicine that can be given to a child to treat allergies permanently or to prevent its occurrence in the first place.

Therefore, it is the best solution to deal with a strawberry allergy, if it is proven that the infant has it, to avoid eating it or being exposed to it in any way, and the doctor may advise giving the child an antihistamine for a certain period.

Strawberry and Banana Smoothie

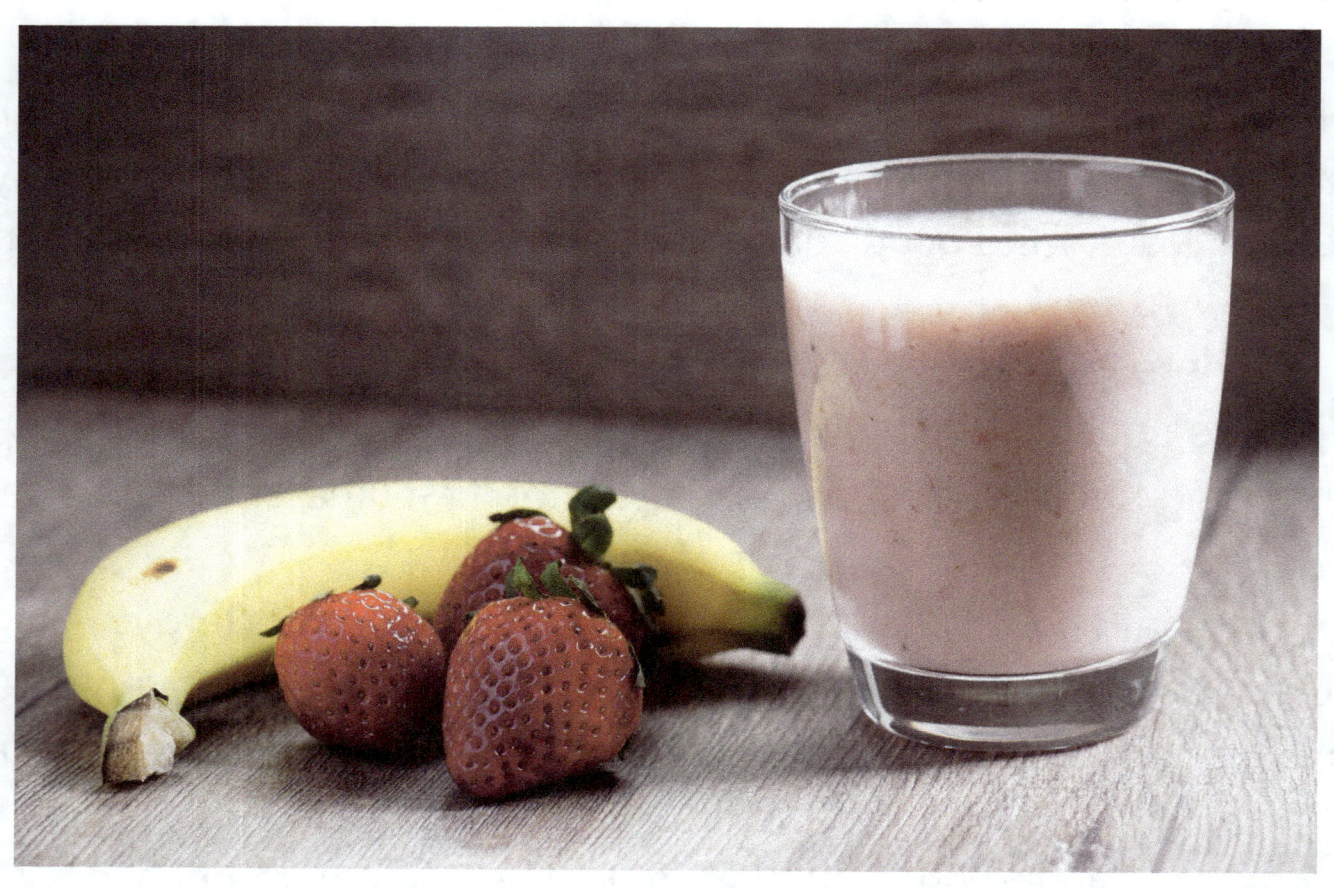

Strawberry and Banana Smoothie

Bananas and strawberries are a favorite of everyone, and strawberry and banana juice is very popular, so what should you know about this juice?

Strawberry and Banana Smoothie

Strawberry and banana juice has a delicious taste along with great health benefits, and in this article we provide you with the most important information about it:

Benefits of strawberry and banana juice

This juice has many different health benefits, which we get from bananas and strawberries, as follows:

The benefits of strawberries

The health benefits of strawberries include:

1. Promote heart health

Eating strawberries helps in promoting the health of the heart as a whole.

As strawberries may have a protective effect against various heart diseases, due to their high content of polyphenols.

It is worth noting that polyphenols are plant compounds that are beneficial to the body.

2. Reducing the risk of stroke

Another benefit of strawberries is that they reduce the risk of stroke.

It was found that this relationship is due to the antioxidants present in strawberries, which moderately reduce the risk of stroke.

3. Reducing the risk of cancer

As we mentioned, strawberries contain good levels of antioxidants, which means that they help reduce the risk of cancer.

The powerful antioxidants in strawberries neutralize the action of free radicals, which can inhibit tumor growth and reduce the risk of inflammation in the body.

4. Reducing high blood pressure

Strawberries are high in potassium, which means they may help lower high blood pressure levels.

Strawberries may provide benefits to people at increased risk of developing high blood pressure by helping to offset the effects of sodium in the body.

5. Regulating blood sugar level

The dietary fiber content in strawberries helps to regulate blood sugar, thus keeping it stable by avoiding extreme highs and lows, which can be dangerous for diabetics.

banana benifits

As for the other benefits associated with strawberry and banana juice, they stem from bananas, and include the following:

1. Helps manage blood pressure levels

One medium banana provides about 9% of a person's daily requirement of potassium, which in turn helps control blood pressure levels and reduce pressure on the blood vessels and thus the heart as well.

2. Helps reduce asthma symptoms

Another benefit associated with eating bananas is its role in reducing asthma symptoms.

Where it was found that bananas help reduce wheezing in patients with asthma, as a result of its antioxidant and potassium content.

3. Prevents the risk of cancer

Bananas contain a substance known as lectins, a type of protein, which may help prevent leukemia cells from growing.

It is worth noting that lectins act as an antioxidant.

4. Promote heart health

Bananas contain dietary fiber, potassium, folic acid, and antioxidants, such as vitamin C, all of which support heart health.

5. Supports digestive health

Bananas contain water and dietary fiber, both of which promote bowel regularity and promote a healthy digestive system.

It is worth noting that one medium-sized banana provides approximately 10% of an individual's daily dietary fiber needs.

Warnings about strawberry and banana juice

Are there some side effects associated with taking these juice ingredients? Here are the details:

Excessive intake of strawberries can make the bleeding period longer, and may increase the risk of bruising, especially in people with bleeding disorders.

Using strawberries in larger amounts may slow the process of blood clotting, which is a concern when undergoing surgery.

Eating bananas may cause a feeling of drowsiness due to the high amount of tryptophan in it.

High risk of tooth decay, because bananas contain sugar.

Excessive consumption of potassium from various sources such as bananas can lead to hyperkalemia, which is characterized by muscle weakness, temporary paralysis and irregular heartbeat.

How to make strawberry and banana smoothie

To enjoy the benefits of this juice, we offer you the ingredients and the way to prepare it at home easily:

Ingredients:

Half a cup of strawberries.

Half a banana, sliced.

Half an apple, peeled and sliced.

A quarter cup of orange juice.

1 teaspoon of honey (optional).

The method of work

1 Place the orange, strawberry, banana and apple juices into a blender.

.Mix them well until you get the right consistency 2

How to make strawberry juice: here are the steps

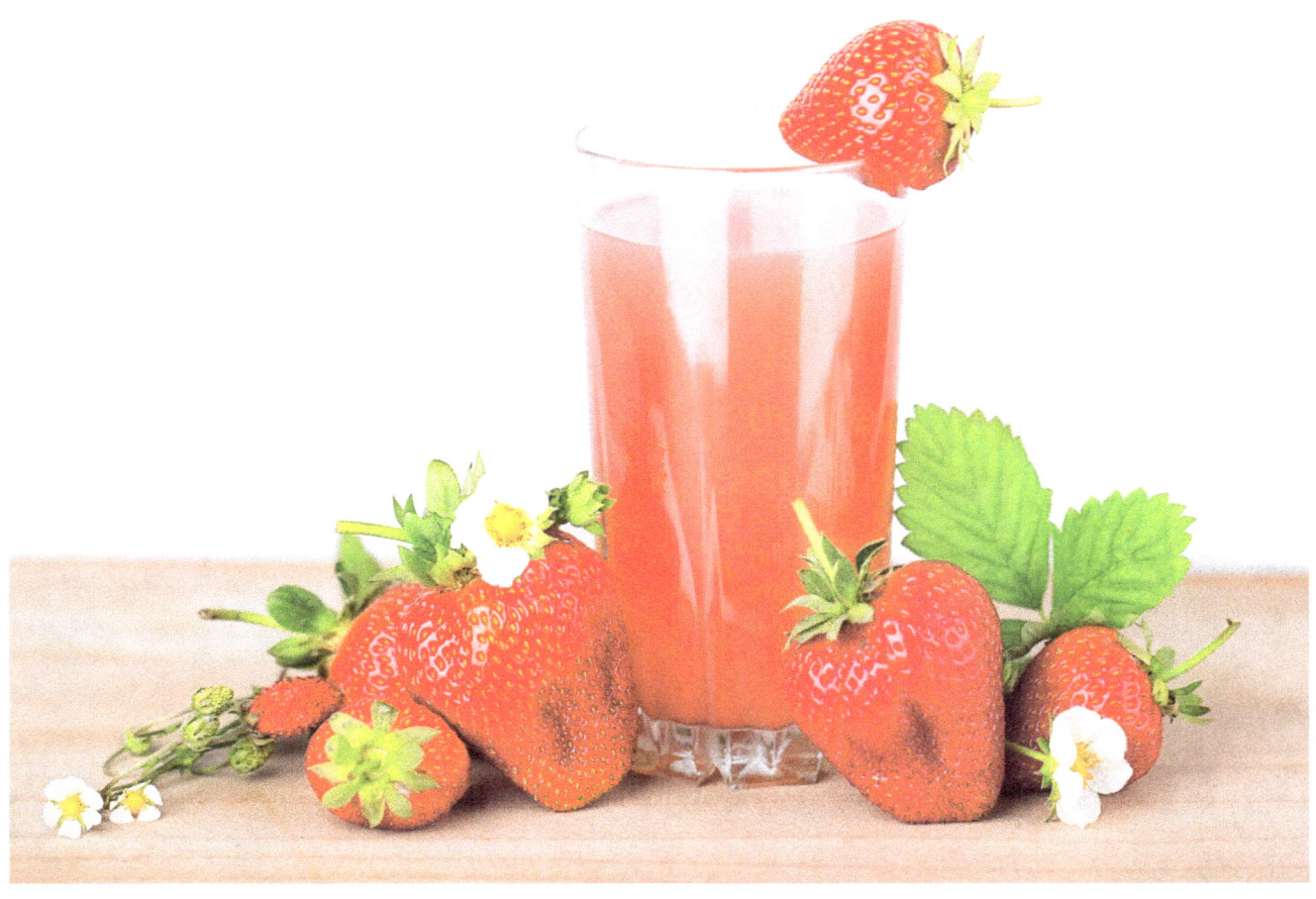

How to make strawberry juice: here are the steps

Strawberry juice is one of the most popular and most delicious and beneficial types of juice. Here is how to make strawberry juice and its most important health benefits in the article.

How to make strawberry juice: here are the steps

Strawberry juice is one of the delicious and refreshing summer juices, and it is rich in many vitamins, minerals and antioxidants, so let's know the following how strawberry juice works:

How to make strawberry juice

Although strawberry juice is popular in the market, making it at home is the best option in order to preserve the nutrients in it and not add additives and sugars.

It is easy to make strawberry juice at home, you just need to follow the following:

strawberry juice ingredients

Prepare the following ingredients:

- Half a kilogram of strawberries, washed well and cut into small pieces.
- A tablespoon of fresh lemon juice.
- a teaspoon of sugar.

Steps for making strawberry juice

Follow these steps to prepare strawberry juice:

1 Wash the strawberries well with cold water, discard the green roots, and then cut the strawberries.
2 Put the chopped strawberries, lemon juice and sugar in a blender, and you can add a pinch of salt if you like.
3 Mix the ingredients well until you get a smooth mixture.
4 Add the ice cubes and mix them with the juice on the blender, it is possible to add cold water instead of the ice.
5 Serve strawberry juice in glasses. You can add a cube or two of ice to the glasses as well, and keep the rest in the fridge.
Note: It is possible to add more sugar if desired, but this will negatively affect health.

Health benefits of strawberry juice

Strawberry juice has many different health benefits, including the following:

Promote skin health and maintain its freshness: Strawberry reduces the appearance of signs of aging, because it contains vitamin A, vitamin E and various antioxidants.
Strengthening bones: Strawberry juice contains manganese, copper, iron, phosphorous, potassium and zinc, all of which are important minerals for strengthening bones and protecting them from fragility and thinning with age.

Reducing high blood pressure: This is because the juice contains potassium, which expands blood vessels, thus reducing high blood pressure.

Control blood sugar levels: As the dietary fiber in the juice works to control blood sugar levels.

Promoting blood circulation in the body: This is as a result of containing good levels of iron, which is necessary for blood circulation.

Protection from some types of cancer: the juice contains antioxidants and vitamin C, which plays a role in protecting against cancer, especially breast.

Improve Metabolism: The vitamin B group present in strawberry juice improves and regulates the body's metabolism.

Strengthen the immune system: because the juice contains vitamin C and antioxidants.

Strawberry juice warnings

In addition to all the health benefits associated with strawberry juice, there are some warnings against eating it, the most important of which are:

Digestion problems.
bloating;
Abdominal cramps.
constipation;

To avoid these side risks, it is important to consume strawberry juice in moderation.

How to make strawberry tart

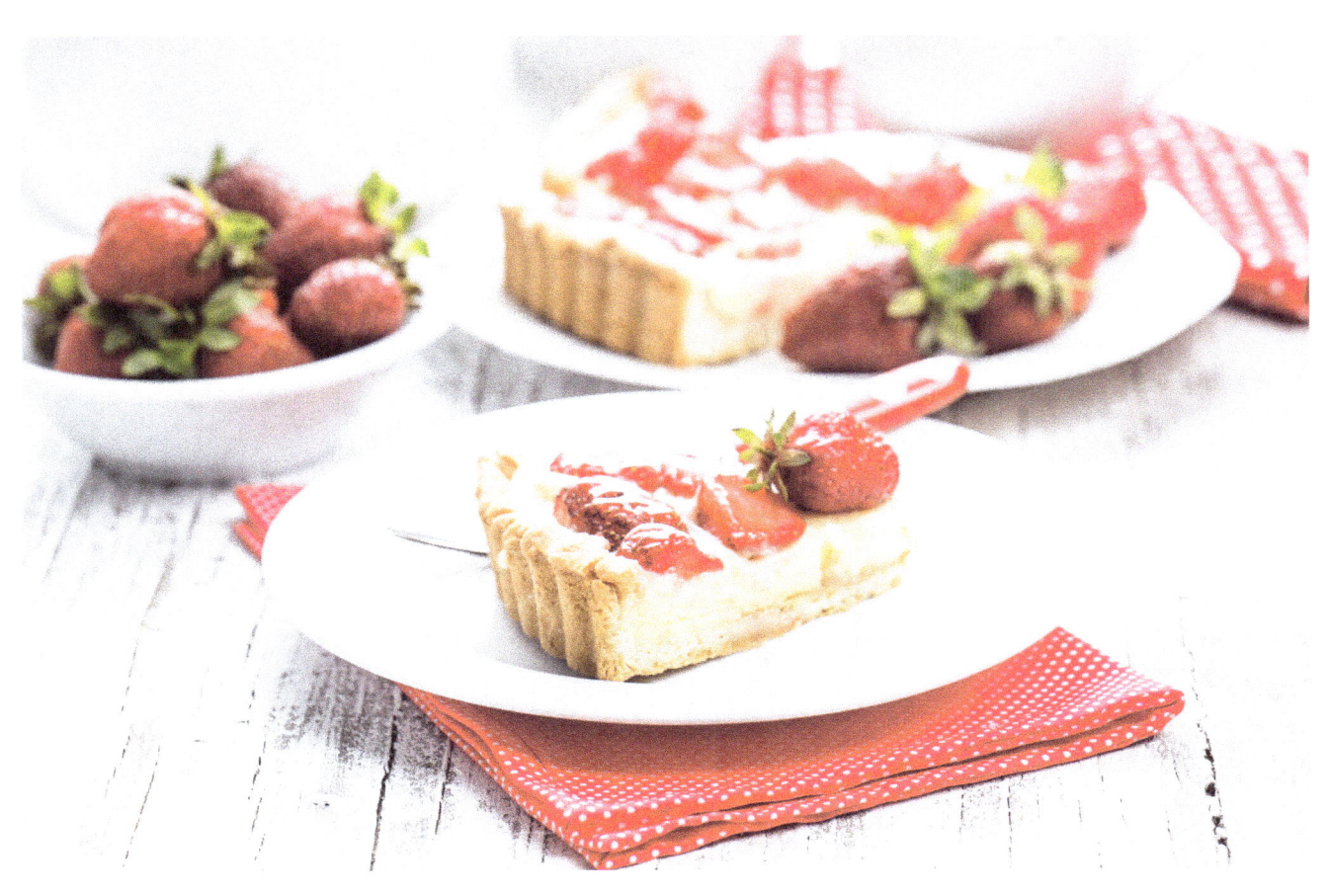

How to make strawberry tart

In this article, we will learn how to make a healthy strawberry tart.

How to make strawberry tart

Strawberry tart is one of the famous and delicious desserts that everyone loves. In this article, learn about the recipe for making strawberry tart.

Simple and easy way to prepare delicious strawberry tart.

strawberry tart ingredients

- 125 g of soft, unsalted butter
- 25 g of granulated sugar
- 1 piece of egg
- 200 grams of flour
- 500 grams of strawberries
- 2 teaspoons of apricot jam

cream ingredients

- 300 ml of milk
- 150 ml of ready-made cream
- 1 teaspoon of vanilla extract
- Yolk of 3 eggs
- 60 grams of sugar
- 3 and a half teaspoons of cornmeal
- 50 g of soft butter, cut into cubes

1 steps to make a strawberry tart
2 Mix the butter with the sugar until a smooth mixture is obtained without being brittle.
Mix the mixture with flour well until a paste is obtained.
3 Cover the tart dough well and put it in the refrigerator for 30 minutes.
4 Sprinkle flour on a flat surface and roll out the tart dough into a circle with a diameter of 26 cm.
5 Put the dough inside the tart mold and shape it to take the shape of the mold, and then put it in the refrigerator.
6 Preheat the oven to 180-200 ° C.
7 Put some heavy beans like red kidney beans in the middle of a tart pan and put it in the oven for 15 minutes.
8 Remove the kernels from the center of the tart dough and put it in the oven for another 15-20 minutes, until the dough is firm and golden.
9 Place the tart pan out of the oven to cool down.
10 Heat the milk, cream, and vanilla in a saucepan over medium heat, while stirring, to make the cream for the strawberry tart
11 Mix the egg yolks and sugar in a side bowl for 3 minutes, until the mixture becomes light in color, then add the cornmeal, stirring well.
12 Add a small amount or the equivalent of a quarter of the cream mixture to the egg mixture while stirring, so that all the egg and cream mixture is added to the main cream saucepan after that, stirring over a medium heat for 5-8 minutes until the mixture thickens
13 Place the cream mixture in a bowl until it cools down
Meanwhile, add butter to the mixture, stirring occasionally 14

15 Put the mixture in the refrigerator after that and leave it for as long as needed.

16 Put a little strawberry jam on the tart dough, and then in the middle

17 Arrange the strawberry slices nicely over the cream layer.

18 Warm the apricot jam a little with a teaspoon of water, and then apply it to the surface of the strawberries with a brush to give the strawberry tart a beautiful bright color.

Nutritionist's notes

Strawberry tart is delicious but contains a lot of calories and fat.

This cake contains a complete set of elements as it contains protein, carbohydrates and fats and provides the body with energy. It is rich in simple sugars and hydrogenated fats from butter, and egg yolk, which contains cholesterol, may make it an obstacle for those looking to lose weight and health.

The red pigments in strawberries that give them their red color called anthocyanins, are powerful antioxidants and are particularly beneficial. These antioxidants contribute to the body's fight against aging and disease.

Strawberries contain an anti-inflammatory acid called ellagic acid. In addition to its ability to fight infections, ellagic acid has the ability to eliminate carcinogens from the body and prevent the development of cancer cells.

Strawberry tart is one of the delicious desserts, but it is high in calories, so it is recommended to eat a small piece only if you want to lose weight.

The cream can be dispensed with in the strawberry tart and just put the strawberries in order to reduce the amount of fat.

Strawberry tart and diabetics

Dear diabetic patient, as this cake is very high in simple sugars and hydrogenated fats that may harm your health, it is preferable for you not to eat this cake and avoid it, or eat a few of it in proportion to your blood sugar levels and calculate the allowed portion of it during the day.

Eating strawberries alone and in a calculated amount during the day is very good for health, as they contain a high amount of flavonoids, which are used as anti-inflammatory and help protect the heart. Because of its anti-inflammatory properties, it is also effective against arthritis.

Strawberry tart and heart patients

This cake contains harmful fats in its "hydrogenated fat" components as it contains butter.

Cake contains a high percentage of cholesterol from eggs, so it is best to try to avoid eating it or consuming little of it.

Strawberry alone may be more suitable and beneficial for your body, as it is rich in soluble fiber that helps lower LDL.

The fiber in strawberries helps regulate digestion, reduces the risk of cardiovascular disease, improves blood vessel function and reduces blood clotting.

Strawberry tart and pregnant women

This recipe may be an excellent choice for sweets that you may crave during pregnancy, but it is worth paying attention if you are looking to maintain weight, since one cake contains 556 calories, so it is preferable to consume only a small amount so that your daily calories do not exceed what is required.

Strawberries are rich in antioxidants that fight free radicals and help prevent cancer. In addition to vitamin C, which is important for your immunity and for the preservation of your fetus.

Strawberries are also an excellent source of vitamin K, manganese, folic acid, potassium, riboflavin, vitamins of group B, copper, magnesium and omega-3.

Calories and nutritional values for strawberry tart per serving

Calories 508 calories

Protein 8.7 g

Total Fat 29.6g

Total Carbs 54g

Sodium 217 milligrams

Cholesterol 203 milligrams

How to make strawberry and lemon cake

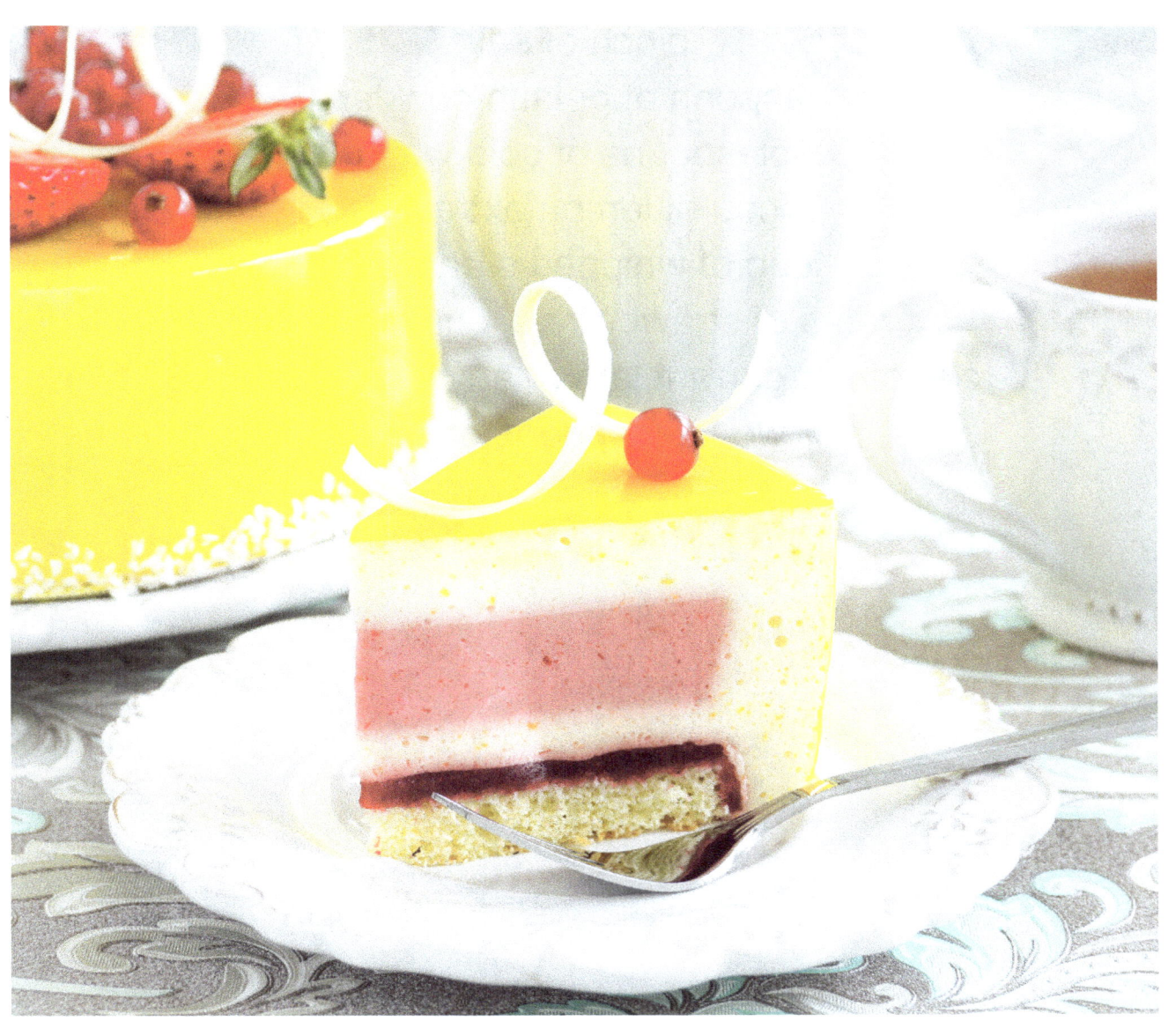

How to make strawberry and lemon cake
- Here is how to make a strawberry and lemon cake

How to make strawberry and lemon cake
Ingredients for making strawberry and lemon cake
- tablespoons of butter 12
- tablespoons of sugar 6
- egg 1
- egg yolk 1
- teaspoon of vanilla 1/2
- cups of flour 1/4 2
- pinch of salt
- teaspoon of gelatin powder 1
- tablespoons of cold water 2
- cup of lemon extract 1
- cup of whipped cream 3/4
- grams of strawberries, cut in half 760
- cup of red currant jam or any kind of jam 1/3
- Two tablespoons of water

1 steps to prepare strawberry and lemon cake
2 Mix the butter with the paddle attachment or hand mixer for at least 1 minute.
3 Add the sugar to the butter for 3 minutes or until the mixture is light in color.
4 Gradually add eggs and vanilla.
5 Reduce the mixer speed slightly and add the flour and salt to the mixture.
6 Continue mixing until the cake batter begins to form and becomes separable from the mixing bowl.
7 Divide the dough into two parts, then cover each part with cling film.
8 Place one part of the dough in the freezer for use at a later time.
9 Place the other section in the refrigerator for at least 1 hour.
10 Preheat the oven to 350°C.
Take out the cake dough and spread it on a smooth surface, and then put it inside the cake mold to take the shape of the mold.
11 Poke holes in the cake batter with a fork.
12 Put the mold with the dough into the freezer for 15 minutes.
13 Remove the cake pan from the freezer before baking and place the parchment paper in the middle of the dough.
14 Place the heavy cereal on the parchment paper in the middle afterwards.
15 Place the dough in the oven for 15 minutes, then remove the mold from the oven.
16 Remove the parchment paper and cereal and return to theoven for 10 minutes

17 Set the dough aside to cool, meanwhile the gelatin and water in a bowl.

18 Allow the gelatin to dissolve in the water for 5 minutes.

19 Put the lemon extract in another bowl.

20 Add the cream to the gelatin bowl until the ingredients are well mixed.

21 Add the cream and gelatin mixture to the bowl containing the lemon extract.

22 Put the lemon and cream mixture into the cake batter.

23 Cover the cake pan and put it in the fridge for at least an hour.

24 To make the jam sauce for garnish: Heat the jam and water a little while stirring well.

25 Place the strawberry pieces on the surface of the cake in a circular motion, or as desired, after taking them out of the refrigerator.

26 Apply the jam sauce to the strawberries with the brush.

Nutritionist's notes

The red pigments in strawberries that give them their red color, called anthocyanins, are powerful antioxidants and are especially useful in the body's fight against aging and disease.

Strawberries contain an anti-inflammatory acid called ellagic acid. In addition to its ability to fight infections, ellagic acid has the ability to eliminate carcinogens from the body and prevent the development of cancer cells.

It is not recommended to eat more than one piece of strawberry and lemon cake because it contains a large amount of sugar and fat.

Strawberry and lemon cake and diabetics

It is not recommended for diabetics to eat sweets in large quantities, as this raises the level of sugar in the blood, so it is possible to eat a small piece only for diabetics and not on a daily basis.

Eating strawberries alone and in a calculated amount during the day is very good for health, as they contain a high amount of flavonoids, which are used as anti-inflammatory and help protect the heart. Because of its anti-inflammatory properties, it is also effective against arthritis.

Strawberry and lemon cake and heart patients

This cake contains harmful fats in its components "hydrogenated fats" as it contains butter.

Cake contains a high percentage of cholesterol from eggs, so it is best to try to avoid eating it or consuming little of it.

Strawberry alone may be the most appropriate and most beneficial for your body, as it is rich in soluble fiber that helps lower LDL.

The fiber in strawberries helps regulate digestion, reduces the risk of cardiovascular disease, improves blood vessel function and reduces blood clotting.

Strawberry and lemon cake and pregnant women

Strawberries are rich in antioxidants that fight free radicals and help prevent cancer. In addition to vitamin C, which is important for your immunity and for the preservation of your fetus.

Strawberries are also an excellent source of vitamin K, manganese, folic acid, potassium, riboflavin, vitamins of group B, copper, magnesium and omega-3.

Calories and nutritional values of strawberry and lemon cake per serving

Calories 506 calories

Total Fat 33g

Cholesterol 192 milligrams

Sodium 294 milligrams

Total Carbs 50.8 g

Protein 8.9 g

How to make strawberry jam

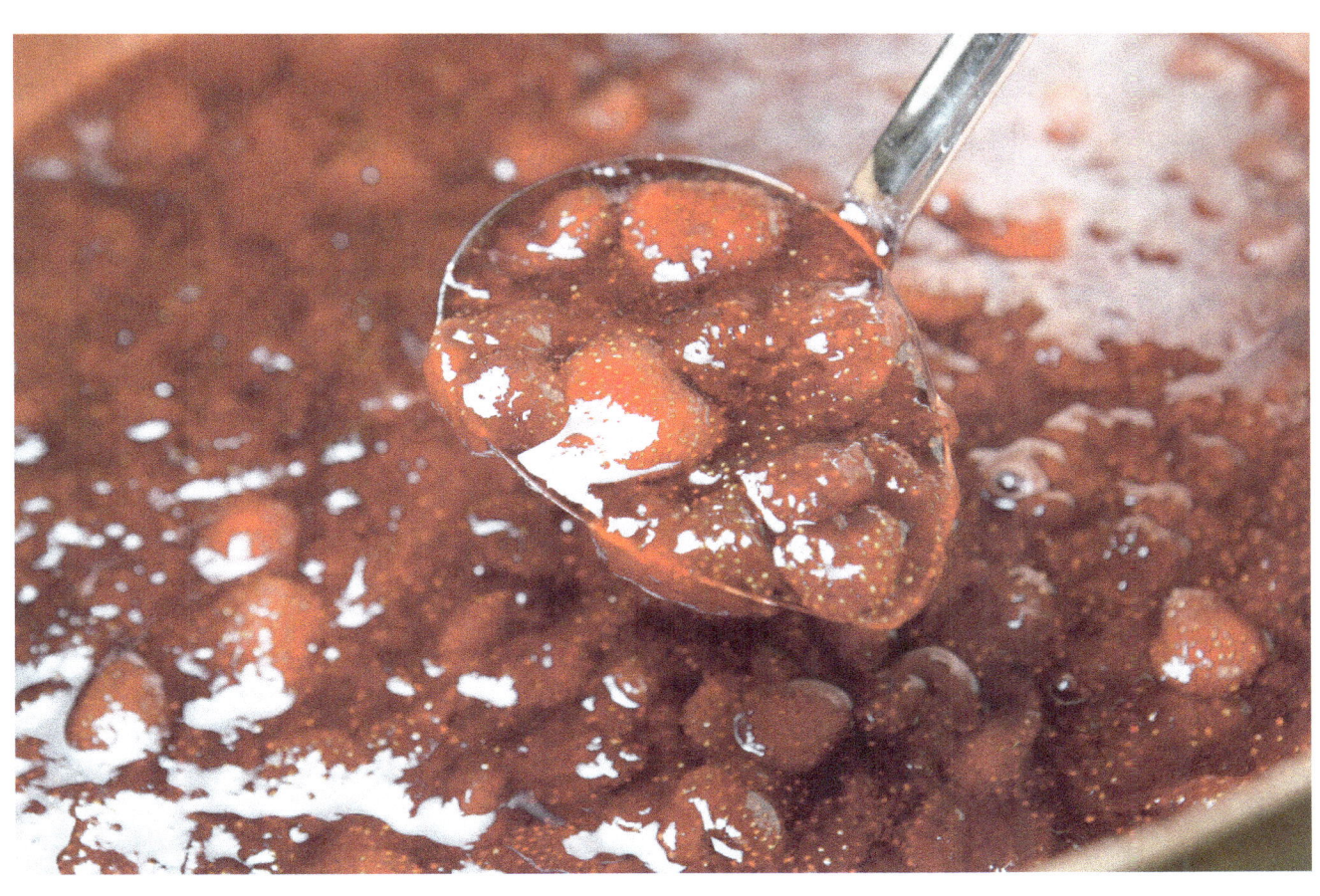

How to make strawberry jam

Strawberry jam is one of the foods loved by many, and some tend to prepare it at home, so we offer you how to make strawberry jam in simple and easy steps.

How to make strawberry jam

Strawberry jam can be prepared at home and enjoy its delicious taste, here is how to make strawberry jam in this article.

How to make strawberry jam: here is a group of them

Here is a group of easy ways to prepare strawberry jam at home:

1. The classic strawberry jam recipe

To prepare this recipe, you need 20 minutes to prepare, and then 20 minutes to cook.

Ingredients:

To prepare this recipe you will need the following ingredients:

- One kilo of fresh and peeled strawberries.
- Four cups of white sugar.
- quarter cup of lemon juice.

How to make classic strawberry jam:

The method of making strawberry jam is very easy, and it can be prepared by following the following steps:

Put the strawberries in a bowl and mash them well until you get four cups of strawberry puree.
Put the strawberry puree on a saucepan with all the ingredients and bring it to a boil, and stir until the sugar dissolves.
Make sure the mixture boils well.
Empty the contents of the mixture into four cups, leaving some space, then seal the cups.
Put the strawberry jam in the refrigerator until it cools.
The nutritional value of classic strawberry jam
It is worth noting that every 100 grams of classic strawberry jam contains the following nutritional values:

250 . calories
Protein 0 g
Carbs 65 g
sugar 45 grams
0 g fat
Sodium 25 mg

2. How to make strawberry jam by pieces

This method contains pieces of strawberry fruit, and requires 10 minutes of preparation and 20 minutes of cooking.

Ingredients:

To prepare this kind of strawberry jam, you need the following ingredients:

Two cups of sugar.
A large lemon, whose juice and peels will be used.
Three cups of peeled and sliced strawberries.

How to prepare:

Now follow these steps to prepare this kind of strawberry jam:

1 Mix the sugar, lemon peel and lemon juice in a saucepan and cook over low heat for 10 minutes until the sugar dissolves.
2 Now add sugar and continue cooking on low heat for 20 minutes.
3 Empty the jam into cups and make sure they are tightly closed and then put in the refrigerator.

Although strawberry jam has a sweet and delicious taste, it is necessary to eat it in moderate quantities, due to the high amount of sugar in it, as mentioned earlier.

Note: Eating strawberry jam will provide you with beneficial antioxidants because it is made from strawberry fruit, which is rich in vitamin C.

How to make French toast

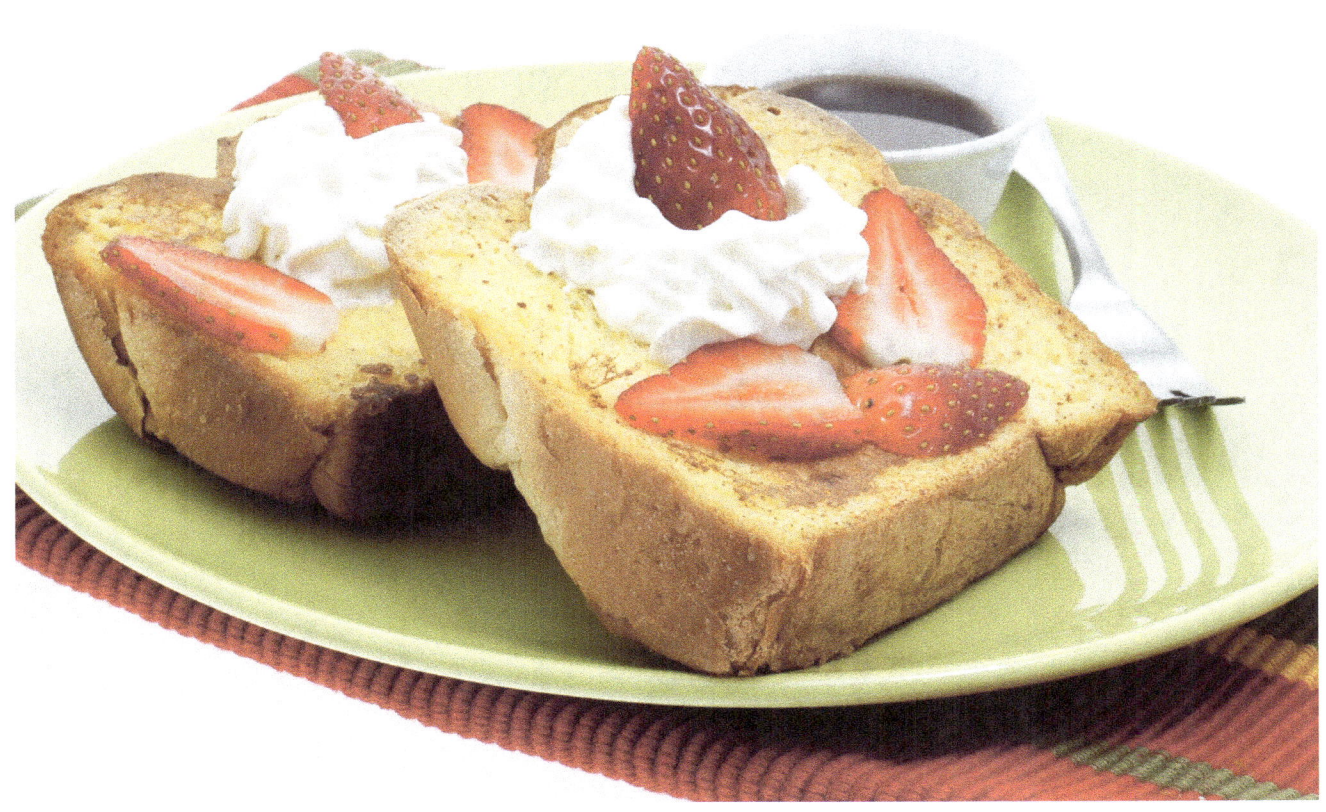

How to make French toast

French toast is an easy and quick dish to prepare, learn how to make French toast:

How to make French toast

Ingredients for making French toast

Ingredients
- 6 slices of white toast
- 3 tablespoons of butter

Egg mixture ingredients
- ½ cup milk
- 2 large eggs
- A teaspoon of vanilla
- ½ teaspoon cinnamon

decorating components
- 250 grams of strawberries cut in half
- a tablespoon of sugar

Additional components
- Maple syrup
- butter

Steps to prepare French toast

How to prepare the egg mixture

1. Get a small bowl.
2. Add the egg mixture ingredients (eggs, milk, cinnamon and vanilla)
3. Mix the ingredients well.

How to prepare the strawberry mixture

1. Get a large bowl.
2. Add strawberries and sugar.
3. Mix them well and leave them for 20 minutes.

How to make French toast

1. Bring a large non-stick frying pan.
2. Melt a tablespoon of butter over a medium heat.
3. Dip a piece of bread quickly into the egg mixture, covering it on both sides.
4. Place a piece of bread in the skillet, and toast with butter for 2-3 minutes.
5. Repeat the same steps with the rest of the bread slices and gradually add the butter to the same skillet.

1. How to serve French toast
2. Transfer the bread to suitable serving plates.
3. Garnish with the strawberry and sugar mixture.

Serve slices of French bread with butter and maple syrup, if desired.

Nutritionist's notes

The ingredients used in French toast contain bread made from white flour, and the flour is devoid of nutrients that enhance the feeling of satiety and fullness, so be sure to eat it with caution.

Rich in iodine, vitamin C and phytochemicals, strawberries are recommended to maintain the functioning of the nervous system and cognitive functions, by enhancing blood flow to the brain and reducing the risk of age-related cognitive decline.

French toast and diabetics

White bread of all kinds contains a high percentage of carbohydrates, and it also has a high glycemic index, which makes it a direct cause of raising the level of sugar in the blood. Be sure to replace white toast with whole-grain bread, to get more dietary fiber that helps maintain blood sugar levels.

French toast and heart patients

The previous method of making French toast contains the ingredient of bread made from flour, which is not recommended to be consumed in excess to avoid harmful visceral fat surrounding vital organs such as the liver and heart.

It is recommended to eat strawberries for their content rich in healthy antioxidants that promote heart health, and they contain phenolic compounds that contribute to reducing the risk of high cholesterol and the risk of vascular disease.

French toast and pregnant women

When you follow the method of making French toast, be sure to add some pieces of fruits to the serving, to get the nutritious minerals and vitamins that promote the growth and development of the fetus.

Strawberries contain folic acid, eat them to prevent birth defects during pregnancy.

It should be noted that the following table shows the nutritional values of the dish without calculating the amount of additional ingredients (maple syrup and butter).

Calories and nutritional values for French toast per serving

Calories 476 calories
Total Fat 20.9 g
Saturated fat 9.8 g
Cholesterol 158 milligrams
Sodium 609 mg
Total Carbs 59.2 g
Dietary fiber 2.9 g
Total sugar 16.4 g
Protein 14.2 g
Vitamin D 20 mcg
Calcium 287 milligrams
Iron 4 milligrams
Potassium 203 milligrams

Strawberry side effects: what are they?

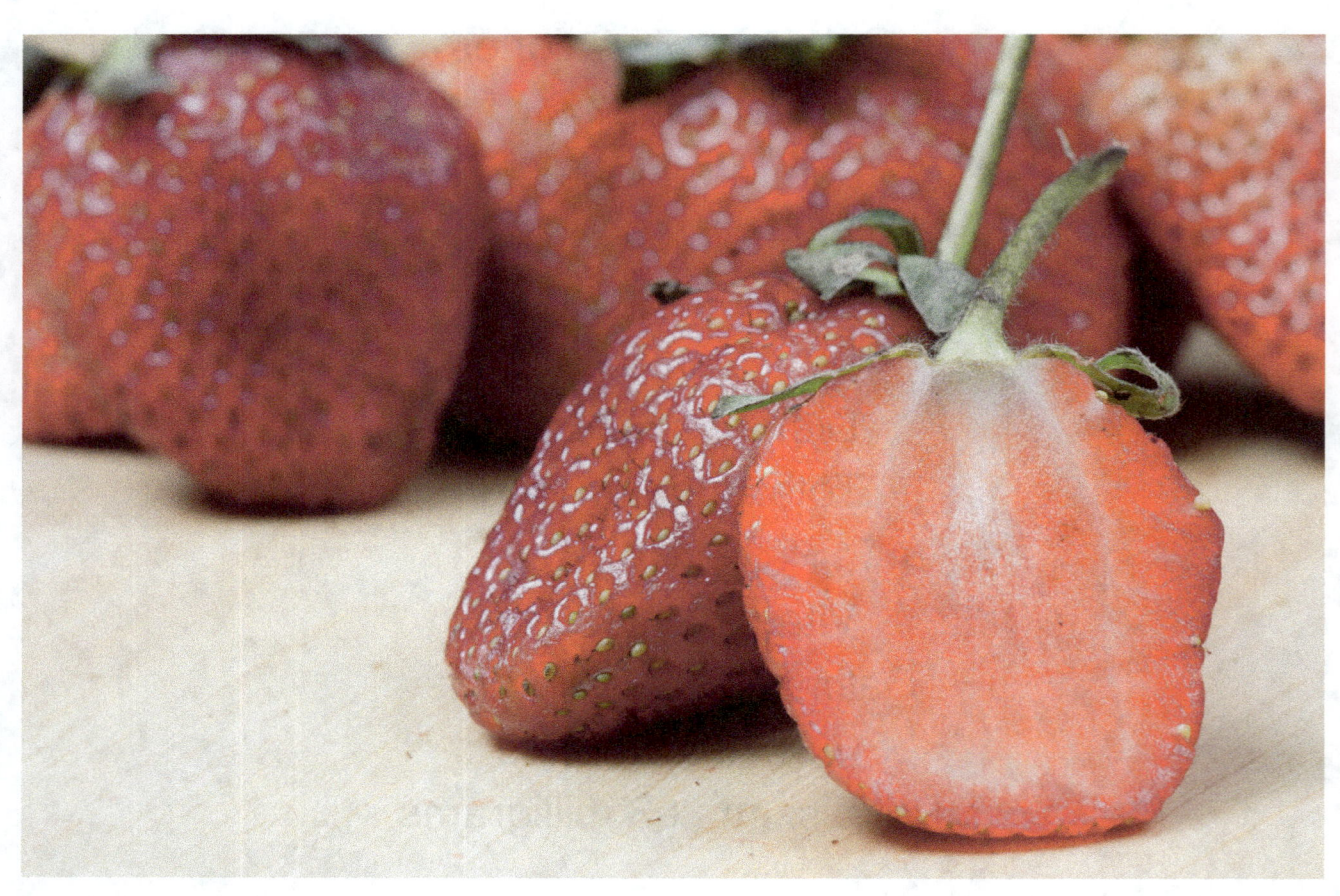

Strawberry side effects: what are they?

Despite the many benefits of strawberries, there are some harms related to them as well. What are the harms of strawberries? Learn about it through this article.

Strawberry side effects: what are they?

Strawberries are a useful fruit that contains a large group of antioxidants, but what are the harms of strawberries? Here are the details.

Strawberry side effects

There are some harms associated with eating strawberries, especially in the event of an excess. Learn about the harms of strawberries in the following:

1. Exacerbate bleeding disorders

It is not recommended for those who suffer from bleeding disorders to use strawberries in large quantities, because they can increase the prolongation of bleeding time, and may increase the risk of bruising and bleeding in people who suffer from the problem of bleeding disorders.

This means that it is important to never overeat this fruit.

2. It may cause problems with blood clotting for those who underwent surgery

People who have undergone any surgery are not advised to eat large quantities of strawberries, because one of the harms of strawberries is that it may slow blood clotting.

There is also some concern that excessive intake of strawberries may increase the chance of bleeding during and after surgery, so it is best to stop eating strawberries at least two weeks before surgery.

3. May contain a high percentage of pesticide residues

Strawberries are classified as one of the most fruits and vegetables that may contain pesticide residues, which may harm human health.

That is why it is encouraged to buy organic strawberries as often as possible.

4. Incompatible with some types of medicines

Another disadvantage of strawberries is that they may interfere with some types of medications, such as: beta-blockers, which are medications commonly prescribed by a doctor for heart patients.

It is worth noting that this medication increases potassium levels in the blood, but since strawberries are rich in potassium, this may interfere with these types of medications, so you should eat strawberries in moderation.

5. It can cause digestive disorders

Eating strawberries in abundance can cause problems and disorders in the digestive system, such as: diarrhea, colic, and abdominal pain, so it is not recommended to eat more than one cup of strawberries per day.

6. Cause allergic reaction

Although strawberries are not considered a common allergen, they may cause allergic reactions in some people, especially those who are allergic to other plants in the Rosacea family

Where this allergy appears about 15 minutes after eating strawberries, strawberry allergy may be associated with some different symptoms such as:

Chills.
Skin rash.
itchy skin;
Swelling, especially in the mouth and tongue.
coughing;
Difficulty swallowing or speaking.

7. Increases the proportion of potassium in the body

Consuming a lot of strawberries can be harmful for some people, especially those with kidney problems.

If the kidneys are unable to get rid of the excess potassium in the blood, this may lead to hyperkalemia or high potassium levels, which in turn leads to various symptoms including vomiting, difficulty breathing and heart palpitations.

Health benefits of strawberries

After identifying the potential health effects of strawberries, it is necessary to note the various health benefits of strawberries in the following:

It is high in antioxidants and phenolic compounds that help improve heart health and reduce the risk of cardiovascular disease.

It helps to enhance brain function and improve the proper functioning of the nervous system due to its rich content of potassium, iodine and vitamin C.

It protects the skin from pollutants and damage caused by UV rays, and helps maintain the freshness and cleanliness of the skin when used in the form of masks.

Helps prevent eye diseases such as: dry eyes, macular degeneration, optic nerve degeneration, and vision defects.

It reduces the risk of developing type 2 diabetes because it has a low glycemic index.

Prepare and compose
Professor / Radwan Abu Bakr
All copyrights reserved to the author .© 2022

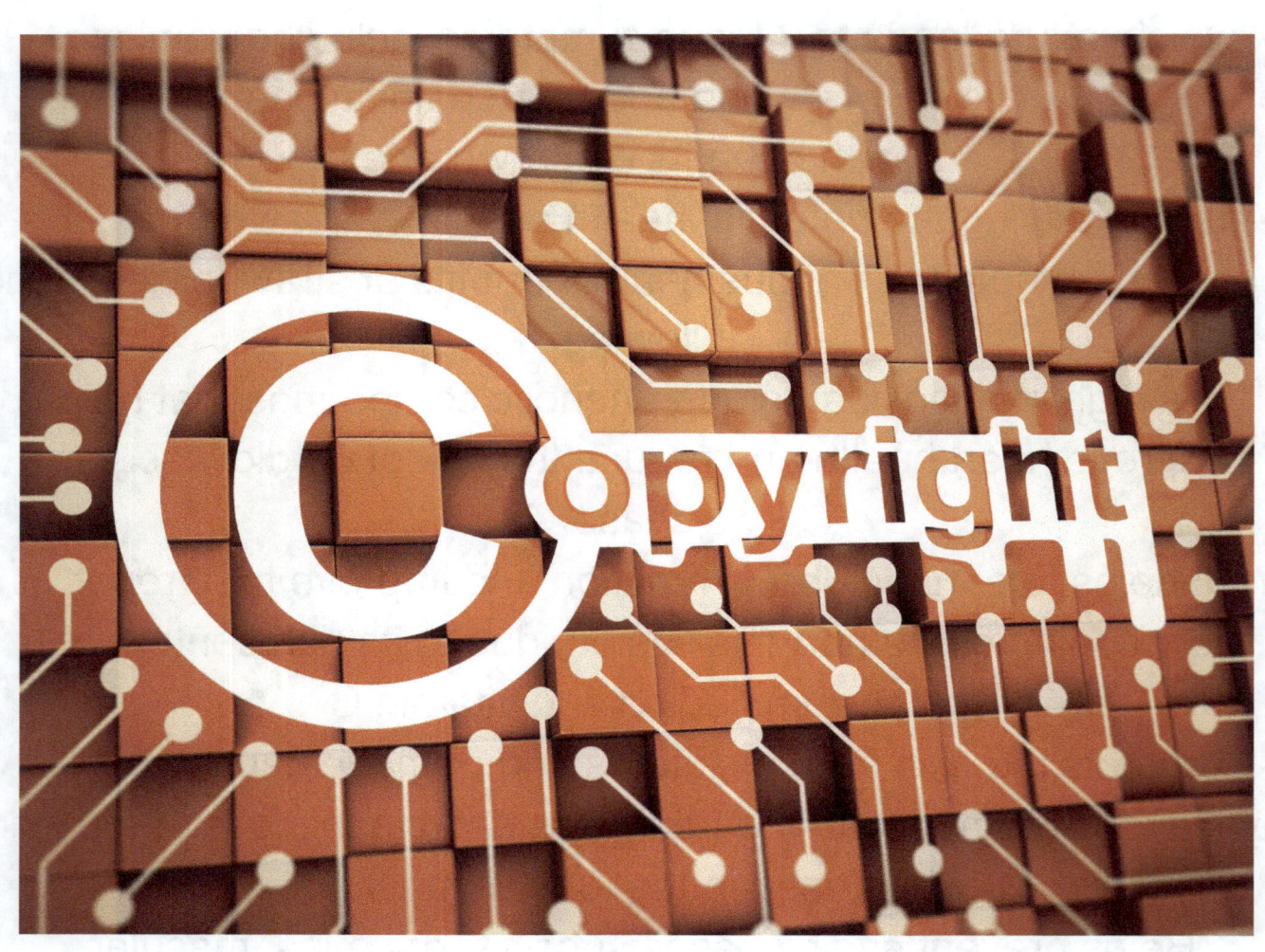

www.ingramcontent.com/pod-product-compliance
Lightning Source LLC
Chambersburg PA
CBHW062358220526
45472CB00008B/1859